MYSTIQUE, MAGIC AND MEDICINE

MYSTIQUE, MAGIC AND MEDICINE

J.H. LEAVESLEY

Published by ABC Enterprises for the
AUSTRALIAN BROADCASTING CORPORATION
Box 9994 GPO Sydney NSW 2001
150 William Street Sydney NSW

First published April 1987

National Library of Australia
Cataloguing-in-Publication entry
Leavesley, J.H. (James H.), 1929- .
Mystique, magic & medicine.

ISBN 0 642 52764 4.

1. Medicine, Ancient. 2. Medicine, Magic, mystic and spagiric. 3. Medicine, Primitive. I. Australian Broadcasting Corporation. II. Title. III. Title : Mystique, magic & medicine (Radio program).

610'.93

Illustrated by Margaret Packham
Edited by Nina Riemer
Designed by David Roseman
Set in 11/12 Souvenir by Midland Typesetters, Victoria
Printed and bound in Australia
0100404-8-995

CONTENTS

ACKNOWLEDGMENTS

SEVERAL OF the illustrations in this book are drawings of historical objects in a number of institutions. They are acknowledged as such and listed as follows:

Venus of Willendorf – *Naturhistorisches* Museum, Vienna
Code of Hammurabi – The Louvre, Paris
Relief of Dhanvantari – *Musée Guimet*, Paris
Statue of Imhotep – Wellcome Historical Museum, London
Statue of Aescalapius – Epidaurus Museum, Greece
Bust of Hippocrates [alleged] – British Museum, London
Bust of Alexander the Great – Istanbul Museum, Turkey

It is a pleasure to thank Nina Riemer who not only edited the manuscript but who has been an ever ready source of help and ideas. Also Lindsay Smith in Adelaide who invited me first to present this historical review on the ABC Radio National Breakfast Program, and Kate Miller in Perth who produced the broadcasts. Not least I thank Margaret Packham who drew the illustrations and was a constant source of encouragement from the book's conception to its birth pangs.

JHL PERTH 1987

INTRODUCTION

WITH A fine turn of nineteenth century smugness and pomposity, naturalist T H Huxley once wrote, 'It is easy to sneer at our ancestors . . . but it is much more profitable to try and discover why they, who were really not a whit less sensible persons than our excellent selves, should have been led to entertain views which strike us as absurd'. Assuming you can handle his syntax, then the tracing of the ways and thinking of the caring professionals of ancient times should prove diverting, to say the least. With this in mind, I have endeavoured to follow the passage of medicine from pre-history, through early civilisation in Mesopotamia, India, China and Egypt, to the classical period of Greece and Rome.

The advent of Christianity put paid to much of the superstition, mystery and mumbo-jumbo in medical thinking. It did not have time for such pious fraud and especially not for ritualistic paganism like worshipping gods of healing. Yet for some thousands of years these gods had held an hypnotic sway over their followers. Their influence was based on mysticism, sorcery and the hint of unspeakable magical rites and curses. Throughout that time span the gods' messengers on earth had been a sort of magician-physician, part miracle worker, part herbal healer. From quiet ways and simple beginnings these wizards eventually dispensed their enchantments from huge temples and evoked gods to aid them.

A number of the gods have been embraced by modern medicine as totems – Aescalapius, Imhotep, Apollo. Some have lent their names to the everyday words Hygieia and Panaceia. The fame of a number of the magician-physicians has lived on – Hippocrates, Galen, Celsus. Several locations now in ruins are faithfully visited by dewy-eyed doctors fronting as supplicants to see where it all started – Cos, Epidaurus, Saggara.

I wish to trace their growth, their mystique, their practice of the healing art, and to see what is left now of those magificent tabernacles which were in full cry 2000 years ago.

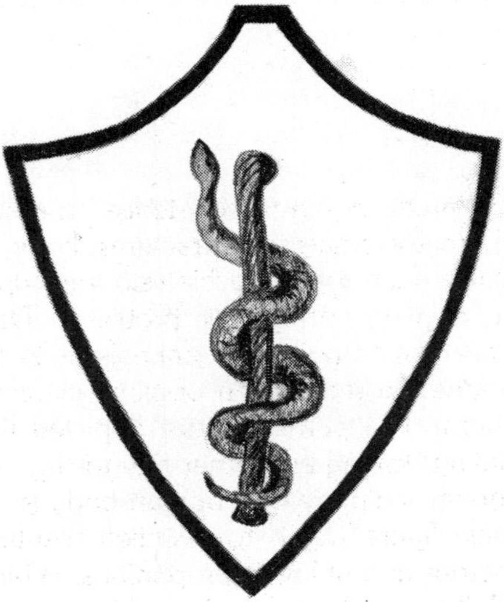

PRIMITIVE MEDICINE

A DISEASE predates human existence on earth. The fossils of prehistoric animals show fractures, bone infections and arthritis. Dinosaurs were as susceptible as *homo sapiens* to dental abscesses and crippling orthopaedic problems. Doubtless these pathologies were just as painful in animals as in humans.

With man came the recognition of ailments and the mystery surrounding them. The primitive artist depicted things medical along with hunting, fishing and other day-to-day aspects of life. The earliest known sculpture of a human body is an 11cm-high limestone female figure which to twentieth century eyes is of somewhat generous and unlovely proportions. Whimsically called the Venus of Willendorf, it now resides in Vienna and is reckoned to be 20 000 years old. It may have been stylised, the ample curves may have been the trend then, or, just possibly, the 'Venus' may have had some glandular disease.

On the walls of the *Trois Fréres* Cave in the Pyrenees is portrayed what is generally regarded as the oldest likeness of a doctor or medicine man. When suitably prompted by your guide, and using the eye of faith, you will see high up the figure of a man splendid in animal skins, striped with paint and sporting over his head a pair of large antlers. If he is indeed a medicine man he displays that air of mystery and dark secrets which some of our doctors show today. He looks frightening and probably was, even though painted about 15 000 years ago. Nowadays the headgear is not too common an accoutrement in the medical setting, but the purveyors of his life's calling are everywhere.

I suppose the very earliest evidence of medical treatment is to be found in the appearance of several 10 000-year-old skulls now in London. In life the skulls belonged to some of our Neolithic ancestors and have been found in Europe, mainly France. They have undergone trephining or the removal of a disc or bone from the vault of the skull. That it was carried out in life is shown by the fact that there is healing around the edges of the operation site. It was done, apparently, with the aid of a sharp flint or similar stone, and presumably without anatomical knowledge. Whether it was to stop a headache, let out evil spirits, provide a disc amulet for a relative or just to have a peek inside will never be known, but we can be pretty sure it produced a bigger pain than the one it was perhaps supposed to cure. Some tribes in South America still trephine and have retained the arcane skill of what is essentially a lost art.

In order to assess how these very early ancestors thought in the medical sense, we can make some assumptions from the behaviour of primitive tribes today. Mind you, these tribes themselves may well have altered over the years, so we must not get too carried away.

There are, however, a few remarkable constants in such people throughout the world. For instance, almost all primitive people fail to recognise that disease can stem from natural causes. For them it is regarded as a malevolent influence of some supernatural being or another human, dead or alive. Thus, a snake would be found blocking someone's path, ready to bite, because it had been instructed to do so by bad spirits. Or, again, it could be the animal form of a sorcerer. There must be many episodes in the ordinary day of a tribesman sufficient to ascribe to chance and part of the grand design of life.

To combat these magical actions there arose the physician-magicians. Their purpose was to observe and interpret natural phenomena or maybe to gaze into the entrails of a sacrificial animal and predict the future with forceful certainty. To help overcome any doubt the magician may have had, a battery of aids came into existence. These included masks and body painting, scarification, amulets and charms to ward off evil spirits and give authority to his calling. Doubtless he had failures so, presumably, these trappings follow the age-old principle that if you can't sing, wear a big hat. Such magical medicine exists today in Africa, Polynesia and Australia, and it is not unreasonable to suppose it goes back thousands of years.

As well as this element, simple oral therapies were used. Local plants were a rich source of medicine and were developed by trial and error. Someone had to be the first to try the berries and both physician and patient would have needed nerve, courage and blind faith. But skill developed and, despite all the theatrical props of masks and the like, the doctor had a real knowledge of therapeutics based on a long experience.

So the two elements of treatment arose – magic and empirical therapeutics. As a result, the medical men of the time can be truly called magician-physicians.

Other bits of primitive lore have become only recently lapsed common usage. The colour red in these people is purported to have qualities which spell death to certain diseases. Red flannel is used to this day for applying to bronchitic chests or inflamed joints in the North of England, or it was in my youth. It had to be red, otherwise it was regarded as therapeutically suspect, if not downright useless.

Surgery was practised during prehistory for knives have come down to us from the Bronze Age and stone saws from the Neolithic Age. Both could have removed a limb with disarming speed, so to speak. Based on knowledge about today's tribes, most of the operations would have been done for religious reasons, male or female circumcision, for instance, or trephining of the skull to let out demons. Trephining was also, of course, carried out on cadavers and the removed disc used as an amulet. The procedure continued in the Loyalty Islands, Bolivia and Peru until recently. Apparently it took about thirty minutes to do in a live subject – about the same length of time as to remove a gall bladder in hospital nowadays. The form of anaesthetic given was a concoction of leaves or alcohol, doubtless used as a supplement to clamped jaw, clenched eyelashes, and thoughts on the tribal equivalent of England.

As we have no written records of medical matters in prehistory and have to surmise their development from contemporary primitive people, the methods used by the Aborigines of Australia are particularly interesting. In many ways they are as close as we will get to medicine before it became a specialised and sophisticated art. I am grateful, therefore, to Dr E M Stack of the Department of Health of the Northern Territory for providing me with details of Aboriginal traditional medicine.

Carbon dating of the oldest Aboriginal remains supports the view that they have continuously colonised Australia for more than 40 000 years, so their ideas make those of Hippocrates look very modern. Traditional medicine is practised in central and northern Australia.

The survival of the local people depends on knowledge of flora and fauna in well-defined tribal areas and the therapeutic as well as the toxic properties of the plants have to be known. Doubtless the development of skills has been by lengthy series of trials and error. One error and a whole family unit could go, which would not have been good for the administrators' image. Being nomadic, like most people of pre-history were, Aborigines do not cultivate or store plants but gather them on the move. So important are they for living that their likenesses have passed into their art work.

Herbal remedies are used for minor ailments. Serious illnesses, as we have seen elsewhere in the world, are regarded as the work of sorcerers, reserved for those who break ceremonial law or as a revenge for past hurts. Such diseases can only be cured by Ngangkari, a medicine man with special healing powers and an ability to communicate with evil spirits. The translation of an individual to such a singular position is by collective tribal decision.

All tribal Aborigines are knowledgeable about commonly used medicines but limit themselves to the use of plants within the confines of their wandering. They do not recognise those outside this area as being of therapeutic value. Oddly enough, the same plant, growing in two different tribal grounds, is often used medicinally in completely separate ways. Again, different parts

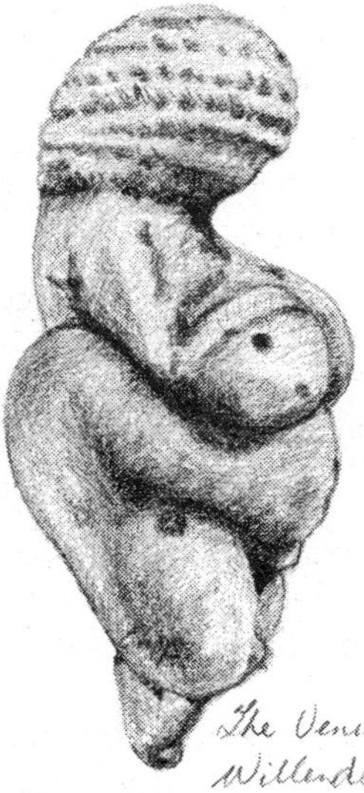

The Venus of Willendorf.

of the same plant are considered to be more effective by one group than by another.

It is recognised that the shrubs and leaves have different chemical contents and therefore have changed therapeutic effects at various times in their maturation. Further, their collection is even more ritualistic. Special songs are sung and traditional paths followed when they are gathered in order to maintain their special powers.

There are specific forms of therapy in existence. For instance, foreign bodies in the eye are removed by squirting water from a well-filled mouth into the offending orbit. Toothache from a hollow molar is seen off by the insertion of a heated twig into the hole. I am not sure that sometimes the treatment is not worse than the complaint.

Well-tried mixtures are used in certain conditions. White clay, akin to our kaolin, is given for diarrhoea. Ochre promotes wound healing and if mixed with goanna fat is excellent for burns. It is only effective, of course, if application is accompanied by the appropriate song. Eucalyptus gum is also used for wounds. Acne is treated with powdered cuttlefish being vigorously rubbed into the skin. The warmed nest of the green ant is applied to the forehead for headache. More than that it has been found to be useful in snake bites, abdominal pain and sore mouth. It almost seems to be the elixir to cure all ills and may be worth a closer scientific examination. After all, the locals have clinical trials stretching back over several thousand years and we make far too little of their undoubted expertise.

Such testings are beginning to be undertaken in other countries where aboriginal ideas still abound, and, as could be anticipated, surprising and fascinating results have been forthcoming. Recently, in Kenya, a series of medical trials has been launched to investigate various plant extracts used in African folk medicine. The first problem that had to be faced was to overcome the secrecy of the traditional healers. The scientists, too, felt honour bound to respect the cryptic nature of the old ways. I suppose they feared being turned into frogs. Hence, although there is plenty of material, progress may be circumspect and results more to do with bargaining expertise than with scientific acumen.

The University of Dakar in Senegal, West Africa, has already produced a cough mixture, based on the indigenous gueira plant, which has proved to be more effective than the well-tried codeine-based drugs from Western culture. More than that, it is manufactured at less than half the price.

In Madras, India, a compound recently extracted from the root of the local *Plumbago zeylanica* plant has been found to reduce malignant tumours in rats by seventy per cent.

In Asuncion, Paraguay, the National University has identified more than 200 medically potent compounds used in folk remedies and clinical trials are proceeding.

So there is global recognition of time-honoured mixtures and although the incantations and mystical hand signs have been quietly dropped, examination of the basic chemistry is proving very fruitful.

The aborigines in various continents went along similar paths to develop their own caring discipline. We do not know when or where it was first decided to invest the healing arts entirely in the hands of a specialist, but by the time mankind had reached the stage of being civilised, the doctor was already in practice and the assorted attendant gods were beginning to take shape.

MESOPOTAMIAN MEDICINE

AFTER A long period of prehistory, stretching back at least 40 000 years in Australia alone, along came writing. Up to that sublime moment, the development of which in itself no doubt occupied many generations, we have no definite record of human activity, just intelligent guesswork. During the last glacial age, the greater part of Europe, Asia and America was extraordinarily cold and it is logical to think that the first civilization would be developed in areas where a more temperate climate existed, where the soil was more fertile and where life generally was easier. Kenneth Clarke defined civilization as embracing a sense of permanency allowing men and women to consciously look back and record for future generations by means of art in its many forms, feelings, aspirations and activities of the present. To this end, the capacity to write is a central requirement and writing occurred first in the area between the rivers Tigris and Euphrates, in the Middle East, with records going back to about 4000 BC.

The area is now called Mesopotamia, which literally means 'between rivers', and it was here also the first tentative steps in the field of organised medicine took place.

The life of the people was largely pastoral and depended on flooding, the sun, wind and other natural phenomena. So their

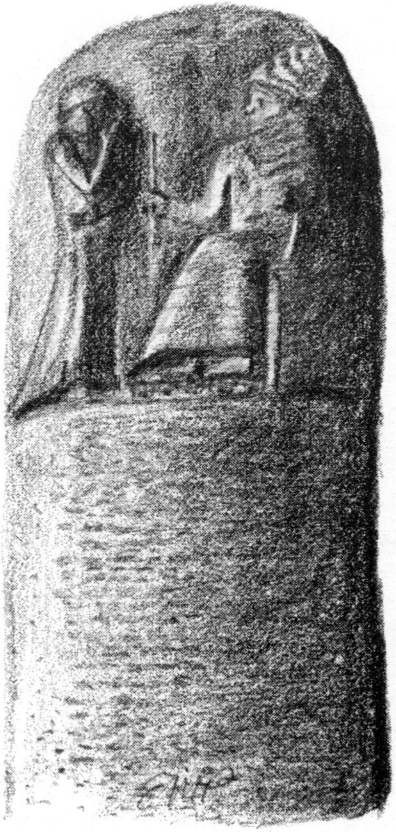

Code of Hammurabi

The kingdom of Sumer and Akkad came to an end and along with its glorious culture the country passed to the citizens of Babylon in the Chaldean empire to the south, and the Assyrians with their capital of Nineveh in the north. The government was a powerful monarchy but medicine was entirely in the hands of the priests.

The most ancient God of Mesopotamia was Sin, and one of his celestial duties was to govern the growth of medicinal herbs. Strangely, these were not permitted to be exposed to the sun, for they had the supposed capacity to destroy demons and had to be picked by moonlight. Secret signs and evil prophecies fundamental beliefs were based on sun and water worship, and their medicinal views were to do with magic, priests and astronomy. The intimate union and harmony between man, plants and animals was a salient feature of life and a cosy arrangement in tune with the times.

The first people in the area were the Sumerians. They were supplanted in about 2500 BC by the Akkadians, but in their time developed not only cities, a form of transport with wheeled vehicles, irrigation, clock dials and copper utensils, but also cuneiform writing on clay tablets. Among the thousands of these tablets since found, some dealt with medical problems. The writing was a mixture of figures and words arranged in vertical lines proceeding from right to left. Representation of parts of the body to indicate single words was common; the breast and abdomen were combined to indicate a pregnant woman, for instance. It was all rather homely.

One series of twelve tablets gives details of a number of remedies of magic medicine and rather laconically begins, 'When the conjurer enters the house of the sick one . . .'. A book made up of twenty-five tablets dealing with obstetrics has also been unearthed. Many of the tablets emphasise the blood as the carrier of vital functions and the liver as the seat of the essential life process. This concept was held by many ancient peoples and was why the liver was examined first in sacrificial animals.

Other tablets purported to interpret dreams and contained prescriptions against evil spirits, most of which had symbolic value. Thus, river bathing, incantations, the binding of patients during prayers and the scattering of grains of wheat all get a mention. dominated the medical scene and Marduk, god of healing to the Babylonians, was also Lord of the magicians. Many of his incantations have come down to us, and it is difficult to say which are to do with medicine and which with witchcraft.

It was in Babylon that the regulations for medical practice were first drawn up and the inscribed original survives to this day in the Louvre, Paris. They were the code of Hammurabi and he had them engraved on a pillar of stone set in the temple of Babylon. If your mind wandered to more secular thoughts during a tedious service, then you could read the royal etchings.

They were laid down in about 1900 BC and were pretty strict. One states, 'If the doctor shall open an abscess with a bronze knife and shall kill the patient or shall destroy the sight of the eye, his hands shall be cut off'. It makes our current medical litigation problem seem pretty insignificant. If it was a slave who died, then the doctor only had to replace him with another.

Fees were similarly listed. 'If the doctor shall treat a gentleman and open an abscess with a bronze knife and preserve the eye of the patient he shall receive ten shekels of silver. If the patient is a slave, his master shall pay two shekels of silver.' Monetary comparisons between then and now are difficult, but five shekels of silver was a year's rent for a middle-class house and a fiftieth of a shekel a day's pay for a tradesman. So doctors were pretty well off, assuming they managed to retain their hands.

Toothache was thought by the Assyrians to be due to the gnawing of a worm, a common belief in Europe until the eighteenth century AD. The symptoms of pulmonary tuberculosis are described with marvellous exactness, listing frequent cough, thick bloody sputum, respiration like a flute, night sweats and terminal diarrhoea.

Drugs were mainly derived from plants but occasionally the ingestion of excreta was recommended, presumably to disgust the demons. It would certainly frighten the patient.

The medical personnel of Babylon, then, were governed by law and were skilled in both astrology and herbs. That much can be divined from the clay tablets which have been found, but it also casts doubt on the description of the state of the art as put about by the distinguished Greek historian, Herodotus, writing 1500 years after the palmy days of ancient Babylon. He states that the locals regarded themselves highly as amateur physicians and it was the custom then, and had been for centuries, to lay the sick in the street to be prodded and mused over by interested bystanders who were freely encouraged to give advice. As he put it, 'No one is allowed to pass the sick man in silence'. Such a claim for treatment for consensus is unique in medical history and I very much doubt its veracity.

Not a single physician's name from Babylon has come down to us. Bronze surgical instruments have been found but no cuneiform tablets relating to surgery have turned up. The record is tantalisingly incomplete, but what has been found shows there existed a precise and well-planned medical set-up involving payment for advice from full-time practitioners.

The type of medicine practised in the Assyro-Babylonian times was a direct link with the medicine of pre-history in that it partly relied on magic and partly on empirical herbal treatment.

Barbarian invasions in the seventh century BC virtually removed all traces of the ancient civilization but whilst the monuments were razed, ideas are not so easily eliminated and they found their way into adjacent developing communities along the Nile and the Indus, as we shall see. The legacy left by the Sumerians to medical practice was the translation of treatment from demonic exorcist to priestly and lay physician, the observation of natural body phenomena and the codification of the responsibility of the physician. It was as giant a step forward for medicine as had been the development of writing for government, law and literature. The thinkers who came from between the rivers are the unsung heroes of ancient medicine.

ANCIENT CHINESE & INDIAN MEDICINE

SINCE THE time of Hippocrates 2500 years ago, the history of Western medicine charts a fairly continuous effort to obtain some exact knowledge of the nature of disease, its treatment and natural cause. Doubtless there were many hiccoughs on the way, many theories were wrong and there were puzzling gaps during which all forms of scholarship regressed, not least therapeutic expertise. But all in all, a science of medicine based on anatomy and physiology eventually did emerge. Such a continuity, however, could not be said to exist in the development of Chinese medicine. Its history evolved along different and unfamiliar, but none the less effective, pathways.

This is not surprising when you consider that the country was generally untroubled by Western practitioners until early in the seventeenth century AD when Jesuit priests trained in medicine and physicians employed by the East India Company extended their various activities into China. If the teaching of Hippocrates and his contemporaries seems strange, that of the early Chinese is even more remote. It did share one feature with the halting progress of European medicine in that after a brilliant start, about 3000 BC, and development of excellent treating methods and keenly honed observation, it went into a kind of recess in about AD 1000. There was an arrest of progress in the arts and sciences, including medicine, just as in the European Dark Ages.

But back to the early thinking of these alleged inscrutable people: let us look at the philosophy which dominated their life including their medicine.

The ancient Chinese were not into all that Western fiddle faddle about the universe being either divinely or mythologically created. They thought, and who are we to say otherwise, that the Creation was generated by an interplay of nature which produced a division in the substance of the earth into two parts, basically a heavier and a lighter. This dual power was designated the Yin and the Yang which literally means 'the shady side of the hill' for Yin, and 'the sunny side of the hill' for Yang. Being primordial elements of the universe, they were endowed with elemental qualities related to the duality, qualities which ran through everything without exception. So Yang refers to sun, dry, warm, daylight, heaven, life and so on, and Yin embraces moon, earth, night, water, cold, wet, death and so forth. Rather cheekily, Yang refers to man, and Yin to woman. They may have known something which has escaped us.

Now the ultimate principle governing the universe was something again and was known as 'Tao', or 'the way'. Life itself depended on the harmony of these three fundamentals, medicine and disease no less than anything else. If you followed with modesty and moderation the Tao, then, it was said, you would be impervious to disease. To ignore the Tao was to fly in the face of the rational law of the universe. Upset the Yin and Yang and illness followed as night followed day. In a population so imbued with these ideas, it is difficult to conceive that anyone would chance his luck and so illness, theoretically at least, should have been rare. We know that is not so.

Another element to confuse the artless simplicity of life was the philosophy of five. This number had great meaning and worked in tandem with the Yin and Yang. Hence there are five senses, five colours, five tastes, and, in medicine, five important internal organs – the heart, the liver, the lungs, the kidneys and the spleen. Each of these organs corresponds to a plant, colour, season and so on. It also relates to each of the others, so the heart has the liver as its mother, the lungs as its son, the kidneys as its enemy.

It was also said the body itself, along with everything else, was composed of five elements, wood, fire, earth, metal and water.

The computations of all these numerical doctrines are immense and can be used to explain anything good or bad. Whilst to us choosy sophisticates it may seem to be too pat and elementary, there is no doubt a brilliant and cultivated civilization flowered under its influence.

But it was not all philosophical adjustments and fine tuning of the Tao, for medical men flourished in their own right and the pantheon of Chinese physicians is large. Naturally enough, there were held to be five legendary rulers of the art. Hua T'o was one who deserves a mention as it was he who was said to have refined the already old art of acupuncture in about 3000 BC.

Legend has it, however, that it was Shen Nung, the Red Emperor who lived about 2800 BC, who founded Chinese medicine proper. He completed a herbal compendium, and no potion appeared in the book until he had tried it on himself. Mercifully for all concerned, none seems to have been poisonous. Indeed, one is reputed to have made the skin on his abdomen transparent so he could observe the eructations and frothing caused by the others. Obviously he was a man of either unique self-confidence or monumental foolhardiness. Shen Nung also codified the art of acupuncture refined by Hua T'o 200 or 300 years before.

A couple of hundred years later Huang Ti (2688-2599 BC), the Yellow Emperor, wrote the medical classic the *Nei Cheng* (Book of Medicine) parts of which are used to teach students in China today. Some doubt has been expressed that he actually wrote it out, rather he originated the thoughts which were passed by word of mouth to be recorded eventually in the third century BC. It was last revised 1200 years ago – but who's counting? He also wrote a text on sex called *The Discussions of the Yellow Emperor and the Plain Girl*. It has a kind of zingy, with-it title, but I wonder who would admit to being plain.

Numerous other books were written in this golden era and included such compelling titles as *Book of the Pulse, Secrets of the Palm* and a forty-volume encyclopaedia called *Golden Mirror*. All this, of course, was while the people in Europe were still in skins and beating each others' brains out.

In many of these texts anatomy of the human body is described, and for once we see that these seeming wonder men were fallible. The descriptions are almost entirely fanciful being compiled on purely theoretical suppositions and natural philosophy. As with their later Western counterparts, dissection was frowned upon, but criminals were sometimes opened up. Physiology was guesswork too, but in the *Nei Cheng* the circulation of the blood is mooted 4000 years before Harvey eventually proved it and got the kudos.

The pulse provided hours of contemplation if not entertainment for the Chinese physician. The human body was likened to a chord instrument and discord could be recognised by the tuned-in doctor. Of the 200 recognised nuances of beat, twenty-six indicated approaching death. The pulsatile spots were located all over the body and it took about two hours to assess them. As little or no history was usually taken, that was the full consultation.

The physician did, however, take into account the patient's rank, economic position, the weather, his or her dreams and those of the family and possibly the depth of his purse. In fact, apart from what we would now regard as of prime importance – the history of the complaint and physical examination – no stone was left unturned. To actually lay clammy hands on the body was considered bad form in a man and scandalous in a woman. To overcome this, ivory or wooden dolls were pointed at by the patient to indicate the site of hurt. A lady's pulse was counted by passing a cord around the wrist and deftly feeling the transmitted beats. What delicacy.

The most important part of Chinese medicine was to be found in its *materia medica*, or treatment. The direction of life was left to Tao, but for humdrum trifles like attempting to cure the sick, medication, acupuncture and diet all played a part.

The Yang and Yin were never lost sight of, so food had to fit the particular element of the body which was diseased – sour for bones, salt for blood, sweet for muscles and so on.

Drugs were given and, as today, were considered more efficacious if they tasted nasty. Animal parts as well as plants were ground up and administered, but the two most favoured drugs were ephidra or the horsetail plant, and ginseng, the man-shaped

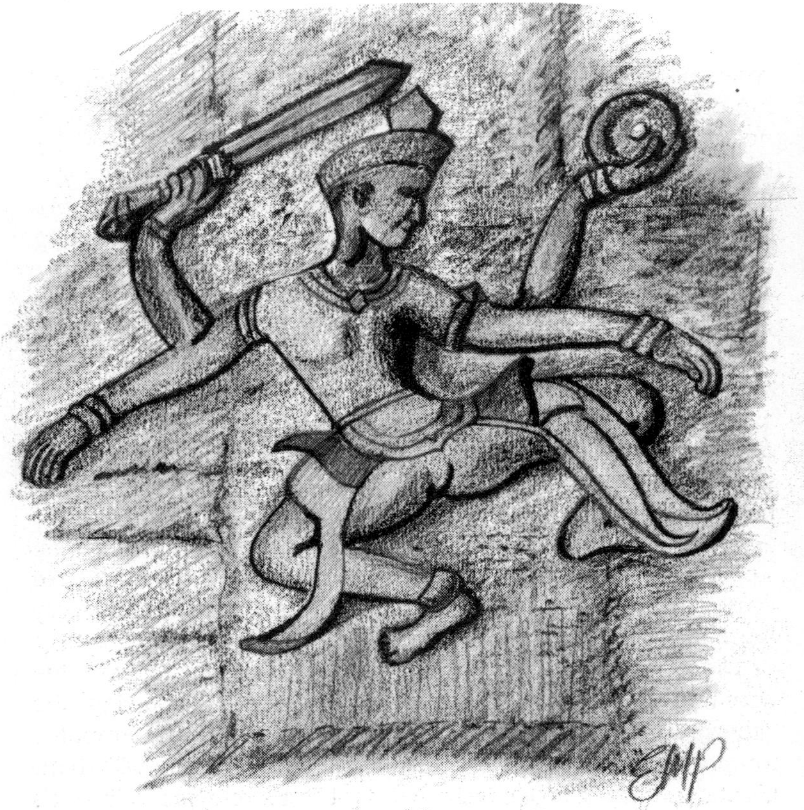

Dhanvantari. Hindu patron deity of medecine.

root. The former was given for respiratory diseases and about 100 years ago it was purified. The active principle was found to be ephidrene and it was given to asthmatics for years. Ginseng was supposed to delay old age and restore sexual prowess. It still has a currency among some devoted and usually laudatory seekers of such Holy Grails.

Acupuncture has a very long lineage and was used to re-establish the Yang and Yin by puncturing the imaginary canals called Chin which run through the body. There were said to be twelve such Chins which were in relationship to vital organs and which contained the essentials of life. Puncturing them removed the obstruction to the flow of bad secretions. Its application has not changed to this day but the explanation has been modified to appease the scientific mind.

Acupuncture was often accompanied by moxabustion, that is burning on the skin the powdered leaves of mugwort to which incense has been added. It is a counter irritant, thus creating a pain the source of which can be seen and which blocks the pain nerve pathway of the diseased part. Whatever the scientific explanation, I am sure it was lost on the luckless patient.

Surgery was a lesser form of treatment and surgeons held an inferior social position to physicians. As with Greek and Roman medicine, the cobbling up of wounds was the major job of a surgeon, but repairs of hare lip deformity and removal of the spleen have been reported. A rather lucrative but hardly intellectually taxing opportunity for the professionally disadvantaged journeyman surgeon to use his bespoke skill was to provide eunuchs for the Emperor. The Court had thousands of these men and as mortality from the procedure of striking off penis and scrotum at their junction with the abdominal wall was said to be fifty per cent, the operator had a nice little earner going for him. In passing, the circumvallated parts were given back to the successful amputee for preservation in alcohol, eventually to be buried with him. Contemporary religious belief was that to be reunited with one's ancestors, one's body had to be whole. This arcane skill was in use until the last century.

Footbinding also had medical overtones as it caused an anatomically freakish deformity with the toes bent under and the foot bent down. It was believed for thousands of years that a tiny foot was the acme of feminine beauty. Further, as the woman could hardly walk, it meant the husband was wealthy enough to support her (or several women) in idleness. It also kept her at home as running away became a slow and tedious business. Only in the last eighty years has footbinding completely died out.

Medical knowledge in China was thought to be a secret power present within a practitioner, to be passed on only to sons or specially selected students. In the schools that were later established, teachers were accountable for the success or otherwise of their students and they were fined if the pupils did badly in examinations. Specialization was the rule and became quite complex with physicians for large blood vessels, physicians for small vessels, others for fevers, massage, incantations and so forth. Always, however, the poor surgeon was at the bottom of the medical heap. Women doctors were known to practise, but regrettably we have no details about them until the first female physician was recognised in the fourteenth century AD – hence outside our investigation.

About the same time as all this was going on in China, that is 2000-3000 BC, similar medical rumblings emanated from India. Phoenician traders sold their wares in India and inevitably also left behind some of the trappings of the civilization in which they had grown up – around the Eastern end of the Mediterranean. Hence such features as adoration of the sun, circumcision, mummification and medical theories found their way into Indian lore. We know much less about Indian practice than we do of its Babylonian and Sumerian counterparts first because much of the expertise was passed on by word of mouth and, secondly, translation of the texts which do exist is incomplete. The written words present as an almost uncrackable code and, further, in what can be read it is very difficult to separate fact from myth.

The name the Indians gave to their science of medicine was *Ayurveda*. *Ayur* means life and *Veda* means to know or attain. The vedas are the earliest sacred books of India and the Hindus believed they were not written by man but revealed by the gods to the sages of the day and then passed on by word of mouth. As this method of communication is notorious for losing its original meaning after only a few re-duplications, then the ineffable gobbets must be a bit suspect.

What we do know is that a magical as well as a rational approach was made to diagnosis, so I suppose there was some Sumerian influence. Omens played a big part in assessment and their interpretation became almost an art form. Hence, if a messenger sent for the physician was dressed in white and sat in a cart drawn by oxen and passed a certain type of bird *en route*, then omens were regarded as good. Riding on an ass to fetch the doctor was bad for all concerned. If, in turn, the doctor met a virgin or a woman nursing a baby on the way to the patient, that was most propitious. I guess the prudent physician waited until he saw the outcome of his ministrations and then, retrospectively, made up the ground rules to fit.

The rational approach, once the virgin had been coerced into crossing the doctor's path, was to look at the result of the so-called bodily functions – sputum, urine, faeces, sweat and so on. Not only did the caring medical man inspect them, but smelt and tasted them, thus displaying a resolve, stomach and fidelity not commonly required today.

Blood-letting and cupping were used as well as purges, enemas and the stimulation of sneezing. The contemporary pharmacopoeia was voluminous and included rauwolfia, used today to control blood pressure.

The Indians of old were renowned for their heroic surgery, though it must have been the long-suffering patients who were the heroes in those days before anaesthesia.

Surgeons were held in some regard, unlike those in China, and had social standing. Operations, especially of the anal area, have been described which do not rate a mention by the Greeks of the Hipprocratic era because they were thought impossible.

Plastic surgery was a well-developed art. Reconstruction of the nose was fairly commonly performed as the punishment for adultery was to chop off the nose. It seems a leaf was cut out to the appropriate size and shape and used as a template. Pieces of skin from the cheek and forehead were fashioned to this pattern and brought over to cover the raw area. Presumably a preferred shape could be ordered and, of course, if it did not suit, then it was the act of a moment to pull it apart and start again. Hare lips were repaired and renal stones removed with nimble ease. Operations were done under the influence of wine or the fumes of Indian hemp. Meditation and trance states had their place too.

A unique Indian medical belief was the concept of *marmas*. These were special points on the body, the injury of which could prove fatal. As, once again, dissection was forbidden, their definition must have involved much guess work. If an injury of the marma did not prove fatal then the doctor was regarded as having treated the wrong site. It sounds as if the physician was on a hiding to nothing.

Two great names in ancient Indian medicine are Charaka, who

lived about the time of Galen of Pergamon in the second century AD, and Susruta, about the sixth century BC. The first-named wrote on pure medicine, the latter on surgery and both produced extensive treatises which are quoted today. In fact, it is said that nothing new has been written since, all others are imitators or abstractors.

The chief god of medicine in India had a somewhat chequered career and seemed to proceed on a downward path, unlike most of his celestial classmates. He was the minor deity, Dhanvantari. He was demoted from position of independent god to earthly mortal, then leech, and he died as such by snake bite.

Oriental thinking and philosophy, including medicine, have a strange configuration to Western eyes, but they suited the times and the population. The conclusions drawn by the therapeutic successes attained by these worthies were probably no more, and certainly no less, than those drawn and attained by the Eastern Mediterranean physicians who were of approximately the same date but on whom our thinking is based. So let us look next at the somewhat more familiar.

EGYPTIAN MEDICINE

THE FIRST really rationalised and organised form of medicine developed in Egypt. Its growth was an extension of the early therapeutic theories of Mesopotamia but it grew away from magical ideas and magician physicians, though evil spirits had their place. The Egyptians organised a system featuring people with special skills who were actually paid for giving advice, the first signs of which were seen in Sumerian culture.

We have a pretty good idea of what went on due to the fortuitous discovery of several different sets of records of much of the accumulated knowledge of the time. First, there were the written records on papyri; second, an almost inexhaustible supply of mummies; and, third, art, especially tomb drawings.

The papyri were so called because they consisted of the laid-out pith of the papyrus plant on which were inscribed the oldest medical books in existence. They, in turn, were generally copies of even older works long since lost. At the time, writing was a secret art and, whilst a number of physicians could draft, more commonly a scribe was pressed into service. He was not just a simple copyist but appears to have been a combination of calligrapher, philosopher, scholar and scientist. Such men were rightly held in high esteem and peddled their special accomplishment in the contemplatively named Houses of Life which were attached to the temples. There they followed their leisured way with no thought that one day they would be replaced by a machine. Why should they? That was 3,000 years away. Their skill was suitably rewarded and was in its way as unique as the skill of modern-day airline pilots, but without annual medicals and early retirement.

The books did not contain all the accumulated knowledge as some teaching was purely oral and given from teacher to pupil under the seal of secrecy. Secrecy in learning was common in the ancient world and ideas were kept so close that, for instance, a simple explanation of the circulation of the blood appears in some papyri, a physiological function which was not spotted later by the Greeks and which was not rediscovered until the seventeenth century AD.

The best known, but not oldest, papyrus is the Ebers, named after its editor. It was discovered at Thebes on the Nile in the mid-nineteenth century. It was written about the time of Moses and bears the date of the reign of Amenophis I (1525-1504 BC). It is not a book in the modern sense but appears to be extracts from different sources, all gathered into 108 pages. The text gives treatment for various bodily complaints, many of which, oddly enough, have not yet been identified. There is a certain lyricism about the writing regrettably absent from modern text books. For instance, faintness is described as 'dumb vessels; the heart does not speak'; heart disease in a patient is described as 'the vessel of his heart becomes faint'; abscess of the lung is 'a disease under his breast like a latrine cave'; scurvy is 'blood eating' and so on. Modern writers have much to learn. Such homely essentials as the ability to distinguish good milk from bad milk, how to improve the smell of the mouth and how to fill the teeth with a mixture of Nubian earth and honey are all in there.

Among the oldest treatises is the Kahoun papyrus from the middle of the twelfth dynasty (about 1850 BC). It was recovered in fragments at Kahoun and was painstakingly pasted together. It lacks the detail of the Ebers papyrus, but does give a fair account of contemporary gynaecology.

Although the Ebers is the best known ancient text, the most important medically is the Edwin Smith papyrus. The others deal with magical and mystical cures but the Edwin Smith is objective and scientific and for the first time we see evidence of the analytical mind. Its contents are based on observation and bedside experience and its writing is clear, precise and contains detail of remarkable anatomical knowledge. For the first time ever the brain, its lining of meninges and the cerebro spinal fluid which flows round the brain are named. A fracture of the skull is described as resembling 'a puncture in a pottery jar', and we can imagine the crazed splintering and depression of the skull. The authors related the brain's function to movement and its dysfunction to paralysis, a fact that Hippocrates a thousand years later could not grasp. The Father of Medicine did, however, quote from the surgical knowledge contained in the papyrus so some facts filtered down.

Carefully described is advice on splinting; applying adhesive straps to bring a wound's edges together; bandages; cautery by means of heated scalpel, and the moulding of clay bricks whilst still damp to fit the curve of the body and provide support. All good stuff and promptly forgotten by future generations.

Now the question arises, who wrote all this detail, who set down the accumulated wisdom of their forefathers? The range is so vast it is unlikely that any one person was responsible. Like the so-called *Hippocratic Corpus*, as we shall see later, it is almost certainly the work of many medical brains probably over a period of time. But against that is the fact that details of the treatment of injuries could have originated from someone with a vast experience in such matters from working at a site where fractures and the like were common-place. He (and it was probably a male) may have been the lone author. A military surgeon, I suppose, would fit the bill, but such a doctor would have worked under pressure in an ever-changing environment and not have been in a position to write with the philosophical contemplation that has emerged.

The man who edited the Edwin Smith papyrus has come up with a very reasonable explanation. Even if it cannot be proved it has a certain romantic and appealing connotation that adds flesh and human interest, as it were, to a far-off and misty era.

He argues as follows. The first pyramid was built about 2630 BC for King Zoser. It was an engineering *tour de force* which is still in existence near Memphis in Lower Egypt and is the step pyramid of Saqqara. It is the oldest stone structure in the world and doubtless its building would have been accompanied by many injuries. Who better than the chief architect and engineer to observe and advise about the resulting orthopaedic bonanza? His name was found inscribed at the entrance when it was excavated in 1925. It was Imhotep, Grand Vizier to Zoser, High Priest of Heliopolis, and physician to the king. The pyramid has six huge steps and is sixty metres high. It took thirty years to build in the period of time when Egyptologists are agreed the Edwin Smith papyrus was drawn up.

The name Imhotep means 'he who cometh in peace' and he was said by Osler to be the first figure to emerge from the mists of antiquity. Such was the regard in which he was held that for long after his death he was worshipped in the country as a demigod. Eventually, around about 500 BC, he was translated to top table and became God of Medicine in Egypt, a distinction recognised into the Christian era. So there is no doubt that, besides being a builder, his medical expertise was recognised by his contemporaries. He was identified by the Greeks as identical to their own Aescalapius.

Unfortunately we know nothing for certain about Imhotep as a physician. In truth, the only certain thing is that he was the first man to use stone as a building material for this is chiselled on the Saqqara pyramid. His exploits as a Vizier or principal minister and architect are also well recorded. His reputation as a healer, sage and magician is less familiar. So, although earlier than Hippocrates, we can hardly make him the father of medicine.

Despite this, numerous statues of him exist, all depicting him seated. Three temples were built in his honour at Memphis, Thebes and Philae. That at Philae was dismantled and transferred to a nearby island when the Aswan High Dam was constructed. It is thought that when he was worshipped the temple became a centre of incubation or temple sleep therapy, a treatment later developed and refined in Greek Temples of Healing.

Imhotep is buried near the city of Memphis, the site of his architectural triumph. His tomb has not been found, but his memory lingers as the first medical man whose name we know.

Imhotep occupied the highest rank of healer, being a priest

physician. Whilst having no medical qualifications, this elitist corps was allowed to examine the patient and take the pulse. The next in line of rank were the lay physicians. They had some formal training as apprentices and had to visit the House of Life where a large collection of books was kept. The ultimate establishment of a University or School of Medicine at Alexandria was a natural extension of this. These centres of learning received protection from the Pharaohs and their senior alumnae were allowed to examine sacred animals, fix the dates of feasts and compose inscriptions. The elder and more venerable members were attached as physicians to the Royal Household.

Many of the physicians and their activities are illustrated on tomb drawings. Illustrations of bone setting, removal of foreign bodies, circumcision and the bestowing of gifts on doctors are depicted. Pharaoh Sahour honoured his physician with the inscription, 'As these nostrils enjoy health, as the Gods love me, mayest thou depart into the cemetery at an advanced old age, and one revered'. It would be nice to think of that happening nowadays. A physician called Nay was particularly favoured and his tomb listed his earthly accomplishments at the royal court: 'the noble governor, the God's Son and Chieftain in the Two Lands, the Royal Scribe of the book of the Gods, the one who is under the King, Fan bearer on the right of the King, Overseer of the Royal Harem, Chief Physician'. There are not too many jobs around like that now, royal or otherwise.

On the other hand, a physician who plotted against Rameses III had his name erased from the doorway of his tomb as punishment. That must have been a terrible social snub.

Only one female physician has yet been identified, Peseshet. As the inscription states that she was 'the director of lady physicians' there must have been more.

From wall drawings and statues, diseases and anatomical variation can be detected, but the most fruitful source of spotting pathology is mummies.

To the Ancient Egyptian, death was a further step in the mystery of life, during which the soul or spirit left and later returned to resume with the physical body an interrupted program. The written language had no sign to express death, just that the Ka had rested.

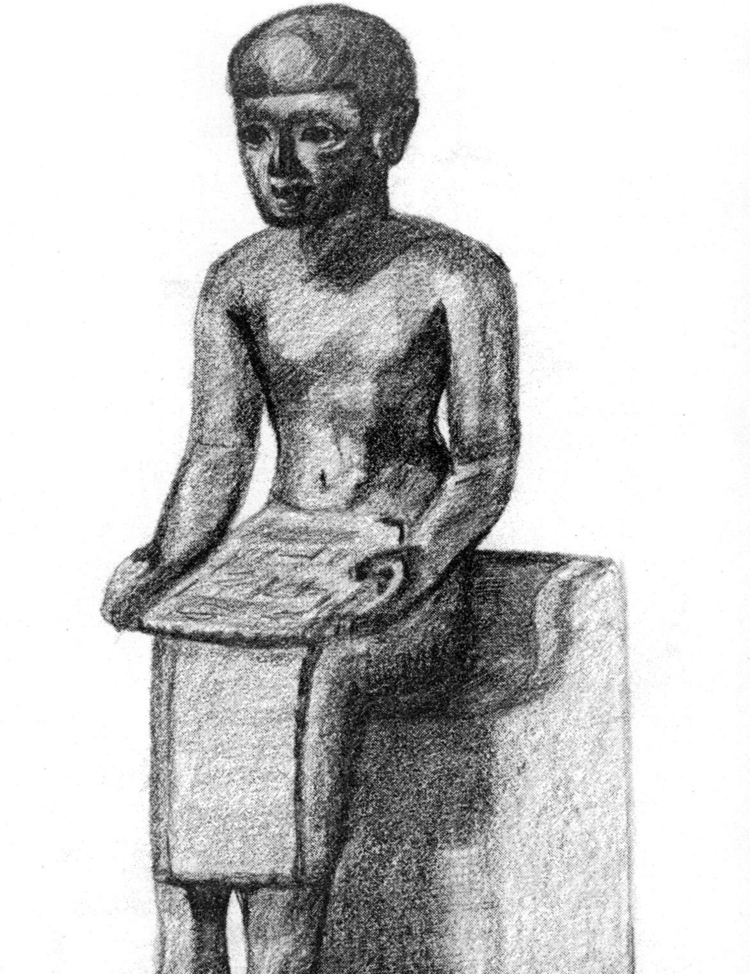

Seated statue of Imhotep.

Hence there was an obligation on the relatives to preserve the shape of the deceased so the soul would recognise it before merging with it again. The ultimate outrage on a person was to destroy his mummy.

Originally the dry sand of the desert did the mummification by absorbing the water content, but later the bodies were placed in rooms so putrefecation could take place, then embalming came into vogue. The bodies were originally impregnated with molten resin which in time became black in appearance giving rise to the term 'mummy' from the Arabic word meaning bitumen. The word embalm came from the Latin meaning 'put into aromatic resins'.

Mummification was practised from the Fourth Dynasty (about 2500 BC) until the Coptic Period 3000 years later. It was at its peak during the Twenty-First Dynasty (1070-945 BC).

If left in the sand the skin of a dead body becomes a baked membrane rather like a drum skin. To render it more flexible and lifelike a substance which occurred naturally along the edge of lakes was used as a preservative. This was a compound of sodium carbonate, bicarbonate, sulphate and chloride and called natron. No details of the embalming art were left in the first 2500 years of its use, so secret was it. But Herodotus, the Greek historian visited Egypt in 450 BC and recorded what he regarded as a quaint Egyptian custom.

The process began as soon after death as possible because of the climate. The body was taken to a place of purification probably on the West bank of the Nile down-wind from the city. Nothing if not practical these ancient Egyptians. It was then washed in natron, so as to keep it sweet a little longer, and taken to an embalming tent. Embalmers were a pretty exclusive lot, akin to priests. The chief was called Controller of Mysteries and wore a jackal-headed mask at certain stages of the charade to stress his god-like connections. The second in command was called God's Seat Bearer and the lesser lights were called Bandagers.

An embalming board about two metres by 1.4 metres has been found at Thebes and it bears a remarkable resemblance to present-day post-mortem tables with their grooves and gutters. In order to maintain the features, the head was dealt with first. Prior to about 1500 BC the brain was left but after that date it was removed via the nostril, a sharp instrument being passed up to break down the soft tissue. The skull was then packed with resin-soaked sawdust introduced through the hole created to remove the brain.

Next an incision was made in the lower abdomen on the left side and all organs except the heart removed. Being regarded as the seat of intelligence it was important to leave it. The knife used was ritualistic and of Ethiopian stone or obsidian. The man who did the cutting had only one job and that was it, for he immediately had to run for his life for breaking ancient law and desecrating a dead body.

The internal organs were soaked in natron and wrapped in linen bandages to form separate packages – the liver, the lungs, the stomach and the intestines. They were placed in four so-called Canopic jars and later left near the body.

The now eviscerated body was packed with rags, sawdust, sand or anything which came to hand, to prevent disfigurement and then heaped over with natron crystals. It was left for forty days and when lifted out was seventy-five per cent lighter in weight, from dehydration, and darker in colour. The stuffing was then completely removed and, as it may have contained vital body fluid, hair, blood and so on necessary for the subject in after-life, it was bottled. New stuffing and aromatic resin were inserted to envelop the corpse in a new-found fragrance. The skin was oiled with juniper or bees-wax and the feet and palms stained with henna. Make-up, jewellery and favourite clothing were fitted and all was set for the bandaging.

Fifteen days were allowed for this, a time mainly used for magical utterances, gestures and other ritualistic mumbo-jumbo. The actual bandages were often worn-out clothes or towels and such like, torn into strips about twenty centimetres wide. A single mummy may have been wrapped in up to 350 square metres of material. The bandage started from the feet and resin was applied with each layer. Last of all a mask was fitted and its quality depended on your station in life, from the gold of Tutankhamen to crude painted wood for the less socially advantaged.

The rise of Christianity with its different teachings saw the end of mummification in Egypt but not before very many people with fascinating diseases and anatomical variations had been preserved later to be revealed to us latter day grave robbers. The embalmers of old allowed nineteenth and twentieth century researchers to have a field day at the expense of their extremely rich clients.

What has been found? Bones, of course, resist decay and innumerable fractures have been detected. Many splinted limbs have turned up, their bindings varying from pieces of bark and wooden sticks to vegetable fibre. Rigid cloth rolls were inserted into the nose for fractures of the nasal bones. The commonest site of fractures was in the forearm and it is presumed they were sustained by warding off blows.

Papyri list treatments for various tumours such as hernia or swelling of blood vessels. These lumps and bumps have not survived the embalming process, of course, but they have been depicted by the artists' faithful reproductions in temple and tomb drawings. Umbilical hernias, scrotal swellings and hydroceles and swelling of the abdomen or ascites are not uncommonly shown. The unfortunate subjects may well have been suffering from *bilharziasis*. This is due to a parasitic infestation still endemic in the Nile Valley. The eggs of the offending parasite have been found in mummified kidneys. Desite all these odd bodily protuberances, a truss has never been turned up.

Trephining as practised by some primitive people, as we have seen, is not mentioned in Egyptian writings or seen in their drawings. Oddly enough many skulls of the era were thinned. The cause is obscure, but it occurred in old people and it may have been due to unusually severe *osteoporosis*.

Circumcision was practised but was the province of the priest and not the doctor so gory details do not appear in medical papyri. It was performed at puberty as mummies of all pre-puberty boys found have had their foreskins intact.

Dental conditions are frequently found in mummies. Caries depended on the ingestion of soft foods and so varied from era to era, district to district but, above all, on social status. The higher up the scale where you could enjoy the good life, the more likely you were to have rotten teeth. Gold wires round teeth to either straighten or fix them is not uncommon.

Syphilitic changes in bone have not yet been detected in any mummies of Egypt. On the other hand, intestinal worms were very common and cited on the papyri. In view of the great heat of the country it is surprising that renal stones have only rarely been found. Bleeding from the kidneys, though, is well recorded and usually was due to *bilharzia*.

The anus and rectum were accorded great importance in Egyptian medicine and several papyri contain many remedies for piles, itching, bleeding and similar ailments. Enemas and suppositories of carob mingled with honey and celery and similar folksy remedies abound.

Eye diseases were common in the Nile basin, as indeed they are now. Tomb walls are littered with drawings of blind people. Trachoma, still with us, led to its inevitable conclusion of loss of sight. Contemporary literature gave a romanticised reason for the disease rather than mentioning the infection that does in fact cause it. The locals thought that it was due to divine retribution for sin, thus displaying a 'Stop it or you will go blind!' type of mentality. By way of treatment, drops of aloes, copper sulphate and accacia were instilled into the eye through the quill of a vulture's feather. Lizard and bat blood was another useful adjunct.

Pterygium, a common Australian affliction, where a small growth appears on the sclera or white of the eye, was treated with applications of vulture's egg mixtures or pelican and crocodile excreta. I should imagine you would have to be pretty sick to agree to such a poultice. The Egyptian translation of *pterygium* is 'fat in the eye' which is a good description when you look at it.

In passing, crocodile dung had an even more evil use, namely as an intravaginal pessary for contraceptive purposes. Doubtless its effectiveness, if any, was more related to its noisome nature dissuading dalliance, rather than as a chemical method of birth control.

Diseases of the bone apart from fractures are an obvious and rewarding source of pathology. Tuberculosis of the spine and other joints, congenital deformities such as dwarfism or club foot and gout have all been seen. Osteo-arthritis, as you would think, was common. Indeed it was the commonest skeletal problem of the era. Rheumatoid arthritis, on the other hand, was rare.

The mummified head of Rameses V is said to show smallpox; that of Rameses II showed he was bald, whilst his consort, Queen

Nefertari, wore plaits. Wigs were a regular finding. King Akhenaton's statues show him to have an enlarged and deformed skull with a protuberant jaw. Regrettably his mummy has never been found and the diagnosis is obscure, but is thought to be due to a rare brain tumour causing so-called *Dystrophia adiposogenitalis*.

Despite all these pathologies the Egyptians showed no great interest in anatomy or physiology nor the cause of death. They just did not seem to have enquiring minds in the medical sense, and accepted life's inevitable course.

Their thirst for knowledge did not emulate the Greeks who succeeded them as a civilizing force. It may be because medicine never became dissociated from religion. They believed that disease and death were caused by some malign influence, probably from an invisible world of hostile spirits, or anger of the gods. Hence only magic or spells or incantation could remove the disease. Later in their civilization a rich pharmacopoeia was developed and personal hygiene reached a high stage of refinement, but even so the supernatural was never far away.

The Ebers papyrus has a prayer as an introduction and it underlies the basic tenet of 3000 years of medical practice. In part it goes, 'I have formulae composed by the lord of the universe in order to repel afflictions caused by a god or goddess which one in this my head, in this my nape, in these my shoulders, in this my flesh. I belong to Re; he has said "I will save him from his enemies, he who lets writing speak and has composed the books; he gives to the physician who accompanied him skill to cure. The one whom the god loves, him he shall keep alive".' The prayer became a spell if the patient added, 'It is I whom the god loves and he shall keep me alive'. Not until the Christian era did that mystical law really change.

So, for centuries Egypt continued in its age-old ways. But during that time other ideas, other concepts and other gods were arising to the north of the Nile delta and while the medical practice of Ancient Egypt stagnated, the new era in Greece began to lead the way and that is where we shall turn next.

AESCALAPIUS AND HIS ORIGINS

'CRITO, WE owe a cock to Aescalapius; pay it therefore and do not neglect it.' Plato attributed these words to Socrates as being the last recorded before taking the hemlock. It was cited in his book *Phaedo* but, oddly enough, in another of his Dialogues, *Apologea*, he has the master philosopher breathing his last while saying, 'The hour of departure has arrived and we go our ways – I to die and you to live. Which is the better, God only knows.' This has a more philosophical ring, but as it happened in 399 BC we are never likely to know the truth. But there is something in the first, and more often instanced, quote which may rouse our curiosity and make us wonder what, in fact, was meant.

It is probably safe to assume Crito was one of his students or servants, but the cock and Aescalapius, what's all that about? Why should a seemingly trifling debt be so important in a man about to take his own life?

Aescalapius was the god of Healing or of Medicine and payment of a cock was regarded then as the appropriate recommended fee for cabbalistic services and not a discount figure for old philosophers of pensionable age. Socrates was seventy at the time of his death. But there is more to it than that and I would like to look at the transaction in more detail.

A cock was a popular sacrificial animal in an era when such

supplication was *de rigeur*. It was cheap and had obvious and noisy life which was easily snuffed out; not a pleasant idea, perhaps, but better than flinging a young virgin over a cliff. Also, it has been said a cock heralded the dawn and as Aescalapius was the divine physician who enabled men and women to see daylight, both had an affinity for each other. Rather a fanciful idea, I feel.

In actual fact, knowing he was about to die, it could well have been that Socrates really intended the butchery as a sacrifice to Hermes, the god who escorted the dead to their ultimate glory. Who knows?

So much for the offering. What really interests us is the nature and being of Aescalapius, still the figure revered by medical people, and the individual whose name was the last spoken by the great Socrates 2400 years ago. Who was he and what was the compelling hold he seemed to have over the ancients?

Well, Aescalapius, as I say, was the Greek god of Healing. He was also the Roman god of Healing, but spelt Askalapus, and he had an Egyptian equivalent called Imhotep as we have seen. To the Greeks he presented in those languorous times as kind, gentle, always available and universally loved – in fact, a larger than life and highly desirable god, a kind of fantasy or too-good-to-be-true GP. He survived in Greece as a deity from about 1250 BC until the advent of Christianity when some theological arm wrestling, so to speak, went on. Christ and his teachings threatened the power, if not indeed the *raison d'être*, of Aescalapius and his followers. As the star of Christianity rose, that of the Greek god faded until, now, one has for its tabernacle buildings such as St Peters in Rome, whilst the other has rather overgrown ruins such as the silent stones at Epidaurus.

The old order changeth, yielding place to new
And God fulfils himself in many ways
Lest one good custom should corrupt the world.

But let us go back from these twilight years to the time 1250 years before Christ when fact and mythology were inexorably interwoven and, to paraphrase Byron, 'when the Gods look on man and man looks on Olympus'.

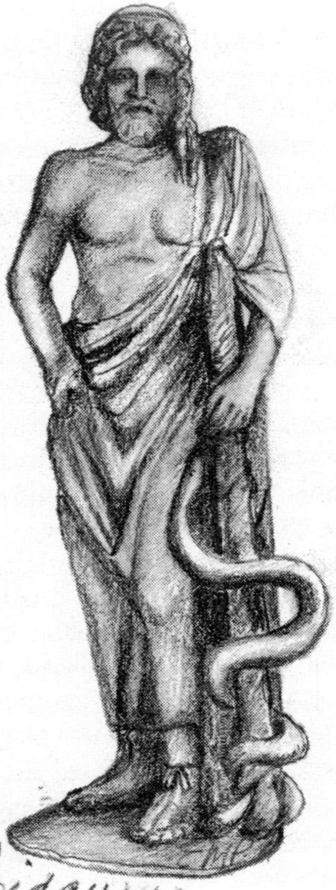

Statue of Aescalapius from Epidaurus.

Aescalapius was said to have been born in the province of Thessaly, Eastern Greece, at Tricca. He was said to have been the result of a brief union between Apollo, god of Light, Truth, Prophecy and, at the time, Medicine, and of Coronis, a mortal. Apollo was one of the original principal collection of Greek deities and he had a twin sister, Artemis. Legend has it that the beautiful Coronis was bathing her feet in the Lake of Phoebus when Apollo saw her and lusted after her, this despite his two professed basic precepts which were 'Know thyself' and 'Nothing in Excess'. To cut what was probably a short story even shorter, the comely lass fell pregnant. No success like excess.

Now it seems that, unbeknown to Apollo, Coronis had been

promised to another and, when her delicate state had been confirmed and a white raven brought the intelligence to Delphi where the celestial seducer had his paradisal pad, the god was so angry at the now unrequited outcome of his dalliance that he first turned the bird black, a plumage it wears to this day to indicate the communication of bad tidings, and then somewhat wantonly killed the innocent bridgegroom. Whereupon his outraged sister, Artemis, not to be outdone, murdered her twin brother's innamorata together with sundry hangers on.

Hearing of the carnage, a distraught Apollo rushed to Tricca where the purge had taken place and, with Zeus-given might, plucked the unborn male child from the dead mother's womb in one of history's first recorded post mortem Caesarian sections.

The child was called Aescalapius. Shortly afterwards he was fostered out to the Centaur, Chiron, an old friend of Apollo. I would have thought he would have kept the child himself, but there was method in his madness, for the god had taught the Centaur all he knew about medicine and the child was handed over on the understanding that Chiron would in turn teach him the art of treating disease with incantations, herbs and the knife. So there was a link between father and son. Incidentally, Chiron was also said to have taught Jason, King of Thessaly, and Achilles and from his skill with the scalpel comes the term surgery, *chirurgie*.

As is usual in mythological stories, there is an alternative which used to be told around the camp fire. The method of conception is the same, but on confirmation of the pregnancy, Coronis followed her soldier father to war in the Peloponnese and the child was delivered at Epidaurus, then a small community. He was abandoned on a nearby mountain, still there, of course, called the Nipple, and raised by goats and a sheepdog. There is no doubt that the cult's principal shrine was subsequently built at Epidaurus but goats and dogs seem to be carrying it a little far.

In any event, the young Asecalapius became so handy with the nostrums that word was put about that he could raise people from the dead. This is perhaps not so fanciful as you would think, because at that time recovery from a serious illness was regarded as evidence that resurrection had taken place after some over-Styx joust.

News of this seemingly divine power eventually reached the ears of Zeus, chief of the Gods. He was put out at the thought of some earthlings being snatched back from his power in the hereafter, so he hurled a thunderbolt at the young celebrity and killed him. That should have been the end of the story except for the fact that, in a scenario so beloved of Greek mythology, the martyrdom had been suffered whilst on a laudable quest for mankind's salvation and healing. Such do-goodery opened up the gates of heaven and in marched Aescalapius to take his place amongst the stars where he remains to this day.

Being up there as a minor deity meant, of course, the heady days of treating people in a one-to-one situation were over. Instead he became a patron and protector of those still doing it. At that time healers were itinerant saw bones, soothsayers, mystics, seventh sons of seventh sons and the like. They now began slowly to unite into a guild or medical association, bound by a common and fallacious assumption that they and their like were descended from Aescalapius. His mindless killing had given them a hero with a kind of *Che Guevara* quality and these simple and good men of healing became known as Aescalapiads after their object of worship. The temples they built to the glory of their paragon and where they worshipped and worked were called Aescalapians.

It is thought that this transmogrification from mere patron of the art to great deity of the science took place during the sixth century BC. Aescalapius then took over from his father and assumed the mantle of god of Medicine and of Healing. He has remained unchallenged until today through 2600 years.

The actual ceremony of deification is supposed to have taken place, appropriately enough, at Tricca, site of his birthplace and temple. The venerable ruins are there today but, regrettably, have not been excavated, so evidence is thin. Doubtless, locked in there is the secret. But elsewhere Temples of Aescalapius still exist and have been located and exposed to give veiled hints of their former glory. The principal ones are found at Epidaurus in the Peloponnese, Pergamon in Anatolia, Turkey, Cos, an island in the Eastern Aegean, and Athens – adjacent to the Acropolis.

One last word on Aescalapius. In his life he is said to have been married to a woman called Epiare. There were several children of the union. Two boys, Machaon and Podadirius were said by Homer in *The Iliad* to have been physicians in the Trojan Wars. Two girls Hygieia and Panaceia have lent their names to modern medicine.

When portrayed in contemporary Art, Aescalapius is usually shown as a mature, bearded man similar to Zeus, but having the kinder, gentler expression of a man who does not know thunderbolts. He is constantly accompanied by his staff and a snake, which, after the fourth Century BC, is coiled round the staff, a motif which symbolises medicine to this day.

The ancients explained the symbolism by saying the snake lived both above and within the earth. In that position it was familiar with vegetation in general and herbs in particular, and had power over the strange forces of the nether world, which affect living beings in a mysterious and magical way. Here the puzzle of illness and its recovery lay hidden. The serpent stood, it was said, for life, dying and rising from the dead. You will recall Aescalapius was killed by Zeus for apparently using the secret force.

The staff was supposed to signify the mystery of plant growth which incorporated the primeval force of the earth. The result was that it assumed a certain fairy-like quality similar to that displayed by the staff held by Hermes, herald and messenger of the gods. As with all heralds, secular or divine, Hermes carried a wand or staff known as the Caduseus. The appearance is similar but it usually has two snakes. The source is different, however, and it is wrong to call the staff and snake of Aescalapius his Caduseus, as some doctors do now. It is all very complicated and the meaning of the two is only clear to the mind of an ancient Greek given to breathing life into such mincing niceties. I wish that was all we had to worry about in medicine today.

But however we may smirk, the cult really meant something to those people. It was the force which quickened their life, and society revolved around these important Temples of Healing.

EPIDAURUS THEN AND NOW

OVER THE whole of the ancient world of the Greeks more than 400 temples and shrines were eventually dedicated to the son of Apollo and Coronis. For centuries people came from far and wide in search of those perennial will-of-the-wisps, health and happiness. They sold off their olive trees and traded in their servants to seek out one of these places. Some of the temples survived for 1200 years and several were functioning until the sixth century AD. Yet again, the advent of Christianity was the death knell of the various pagan gods in the area, but the cult of Aescalapius was one of the last to go.

The Harley Street or Macquarie Street of the time, where the reputation of the priests was the highest and doubtless the material rewards greatest, was located at Epidaurus. The exact or even approximate date of its establishment is not known. By the sixth century BC it was doing a great trade in dispensing cures. As we have seen, it may have been the birthplace of the god himself, but there is no doubt that it was near the ancient city of Mycenae whose one-time king was Agamemnon, leader of the Greeks in the Trojan wars. (You may recall Homer has it that Aescalapius's two sons were doctors at that mighty confrontation.) So the temple was fairly near to major centres, which was important for its survival. But it may have been established at Epidaurus for more practical reasons such as the availability of water and a peaceful surround, the better to contemplate one's navel or one's mortality.

As a centre of healing it reached its peak at the end of the fourth century BC when it became a place of pan-Hellenic pilgrimage. If you were anybody, the place to be seen then was Epidaurus.

Much building took place at that time, including the great temple to the god himself. Built in 490 BC, its pride and centre-piece was its gold and ivory statue of Aescalapius. It was suitably large and imposing, as befitted a place given over to attracting the out-of-town invalid. Across the front of the temple were six great Doric columns and down the sides eleven more. Before it stood an altar and from that a paved road led to and from the sanctuary of which the temple was the principal building. Against the temple at the rear were some semi-circular platforms erected by private citizens as an offering to the god. Sculptures around the pediment were in the characteristic mould of the time and reflected bellicosity and death in heroic circumstances. The Battles of the Centaurs and the Fall of Troy were depicted, as were other valorous posturings beloved of a male-orientated society. All were at variance with the alleged role of the place, but at least comfortably familiar to new arrivals.

Behind the temple was the so-called Tholos, a strange labyrinthine structure of three concentric circular walls. The circles intercommunicated by narrow openings on various axes, so you never knew what was round the corner. The place was constructed in white marble and had an exterior colonnade of twenty-six Doric columns. Inside was another colonnade of fourteen Corinthian columns. The floor was a chequer board of black and white slabs, and in the very centre, when eventually you found your way there, was an opening leading down, naturally enough, to a mysterious lower chamber, what else?

That basement is still there, as we shall see in a moment. Its function is unknown, but we do know the opening was normally covered with a marble slab. Constructed as it was in this way it was obviously an enclosure of prime importance and mystery. Probably it was yet another place of worship; I wonder if they ever wearied of incessant prayers. But it could have been built to house the sacred snakes. Aescalapius, as we have seen, was into snakes for symbolic reasons and so his earthly priests held them to be special, if not essential, in their business of miracle-mongering. They may, of course, have just been there, dare I say it, to keep the rats down.

To the north of these structures was the sleeping ward or abaton. Here the supplicants nodded off, hoping in their rhapsodic sleep for revelations of cure. It was a big structure to cater for the expected crowds, being seventy metres long and five-and-a-half metres wide. Naturally it was a place of more Doric columns. Adjacent to it was a deep well around the mouth of which were chiselled lists of various tested remedies.

All these buildings were in the sanctuary, or sacred area, and formed a kind of early out-patient department with night care accommodation. But nonetheless it was holy enough to have an inflexible rule that nobody died or was born there. There were probably a few narrow shaves in an ordinary working year.

Outside the sanctuary, on account of their profane nature, were present a fountain, bath and library, together with a long, arched building which housed shops and suchlike for the more secular needs of the itinerant populace. The library had a large central room with lesser cabins off and was completed in the second century BC. This was 400 years after the temple was built and perhaps was put there to silence the clamour for some kind of anteroom with literature to fill in the waiting hours. More likely it stored clay or stone tablets inscribed with the accumulated knowledge of the temple.

Further away in the complex was a huge gymnasium, a hostel (or xenon) and temples to Hygieia, Artemis and other minor gods.

Beyond the main site was built a stadium with a 180-metre oval track and twenty-two rows of seats. Round the track short columns were placed every thirty-two metres so you knew how far you still had to go. Nearby was a magnificent theatre. So all aspects of life were catered for, the soul at the temple, body at the stadium, the spirit at the theatre, as well as the doggedly pursued and highly successful function for which it was built – the healing of the sick.

How did they do that? Briefly, healing was accomplished by a ritual known as incubation, or temple sleep. I suppose that by sleeping in the temple the germ of the idea of cure incubates and on waking all is revealed – you hope. On arrival down that road to the altar in front of the Temple of Aescalapius a sacrificial offering or votive was made and a purifying bath was taken. Prayers were offered and the supplicant conducted to the abaton to sleep. The process had been laid down over many years and the patients had probably travelled from far distant parts so were tired. The whole ambience of the sanctuary was one of quiet, almost breathless piety and the Aescalapiads were skilled in the field of quiet suggestion and fostering tranquillity. All this psyching up took place on already humble and devout believers so that it came as no surprise to anyone, least of all the patients, that Aescalapius himself appeared in their dreams. He was variously described as being a blinding light with voice, or an old and venerable man, or youthful and beardless, or even as a child wise beyond its years. Whatever his guise, advice was given, occasionally operations were performed, as we shall see later, and the patient departed the next day cured and rejoicing. During the therapeutic slumber, snakes loosed from the Tholos were said to lick the eyes of some of the patients.

Occasionally it took more than one or two nights and in the odd case the devotee stayed for years in the cloistered and sequestrated surroundings. No sense in getting well enough too soon, to return to the harsh realities of mortgages, taxation and argumentative neighbours.

I will return to treatment in a later chapter to look at its success and examine a few recorded case histories, but let us turn to Epidaurus as it is now and see what is left of its former splendour. The brief answer is, not much. But read on.

At its zenith Epidaurus catered, I suppose, for a gullible and rich population chasing therapeutic rainbows or immortality. Its age passed and to the unimaginative visitor in the twentieth century all that is left on the site is a jumble of stones, the odd column, overgrown inscription and precious little else. But, if approached with a feeling of caprice or whimsy, it is not like that at all. Well, not to me anyway. It should be advanced upon in the manner of our forefathers, with a growing anticipation of something mystical, if not magical, about to happen, so that when on the site itself one senses in some intangible way the devotion, piety and successes of its former inmates. Go and see for yourself or, for the moment, let me take you.

If you drive south-west from Athens through the area of Attica of mythological fame, round the Saronic Gulf and over the Corinth Canal, you will arrive on the Peloponnese peninsula. From then on the unfolding countryside of Argolid is rough and inhospitable. The hills are low and rugged and the vegetation coarse and prickly.

Eventually, in a small valley above the old port of Epidaurus, you will chance upon your quarry, the Temple of one of the largest centres of healing in antiquity. Having driven through forbidding country, along a road 3000 years old albeit resurfaced, you arrive in an area lush with trees, sheltered and calm and quite different from its surroundings.

Park the car and walk up to the ruins along a magnificent curving road lined by very tall pines and cypress trees flanked by oleander. The whole produces a scent the like of which John Betjeman once described in other circumstances as 'mushroomy, pinewoody, evergreen smells'.

Mature and huge as the trees are, they obviously have not been there for 2000 years or more, so do not get too dewy-eyed too soon. But there is no doubt they create a strange feeling of tranquillity and peace, a sensation heightened by the swishing sound as the breeze edges through them. It needs little imagination to feel that the trees' ancestors had a soporific effect on the approaching traveller as he made his way to the sanctuary.

Truth to tell, the main reason for anyone going to Epidaurus nowadays is not to contemplate the snake pit, sleeping chamber and the like, but to marvel at the ancient Greek theatre so, having become suitably tuned-in by walking through the swishing, murmuring trees to be in a position to cast off your gloom if not your crutches, you come, in fact, not to the healing sanctuary, but to the theatre.

While it may be a slight let down if you have a brain tumour or similar, it is at least a sight for sore eyes because, although built in the third century BC, it is preserved almost intact. It is still in use and seats about 12 000 people. The acoustics are so good that the tearing of a piece of paper on stage sounds like the ripping

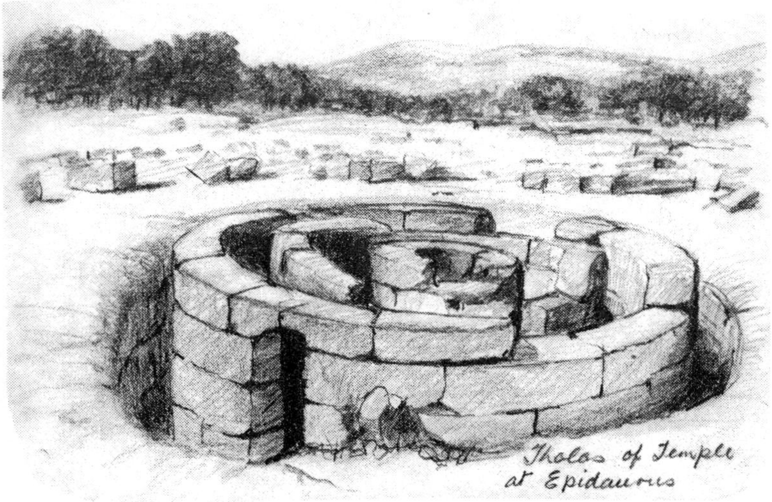

of an overstretched spinnaker in the back row.

Breathtaking it may be, but we devotees of Aescalapius must tear ourselves away, leave the theatre, walk past the present-day museum and into the temple area proper. As you breast a small rise to catch your first glimpse you are again likely to feel a twinge of disappointment. For there, spread before you over several hectares, is an area where it hardly seems that one stone stands atop another. It is archaeological chaos. No temple, no gymnasium, no tholos, nothing which can be readily pointed out. Do not be discouraged, walk down armed with a map and seek out the most easily distinguished ruins, the tholos.

There are very few trees here and it is not the swishing of branches but the silence which is awesome. It is not complete because the cicadas are incessant in their shrillness and the birds contribute but there is no doubt but that the place feels special.

You enter the sanctuary area built in 490 BC where, you recall, neither birth nor death could take place. All that remains of the magnificent structures are the stone foundations, a portion of the floor of the temple and a ramp on its eastern side heading from the library to the temple. You know the strange circular tholos is nearby so you turn and at once its obvious presence makes you feel on safer ground. Because right there in the prescribed spot are the concentric stone walls. It is only the basement, the area beneath the black and white marble floor, not one bit of which is in evidence. Nor is the marble slate which covered the innermost circular compartment. But the three curving walls are there with their concentric openings. The white marble is gone and only the under-base of ashlar blocks remains to retain the air of unresolved and timeless ritual. It is twenty-two metres in diameter and could have housed an awful lot of sacred serpents which could have licked countless eyes or killed myriad rats.

To the north is seen a fragment of a solitary column; at least here there are two or three stones on top of one another. Beside it are several stone bases of columns and you realise that that represents the sum total of the abaton where the supplicants slept and communicated with Aescalapius himself. Imagination is needed here, but to the finely-tuned visitor the droning cicadas do, indeed, induce a certain drowsiness. Or was that the heat, or the wine we had for lunch, or just a figment of a vivid imagination?

You can wander from the sanctuary to the more mundane area of shops, fountains and lesser temples. It is impossible to distinguish one from another and after contemplation of the tholos and letting your imagination run riot there is little reserve left for attempting a conceptual reconstruction. So return to the car and make your way back to Athens, noise and reality.

But if you are reluctant to abandon forever the feel of the place, you have one last chance to indulge your whimsy. Go to the National Archaeological Museum in Athens and visit the Epidaurus room. A number of sculptures have survived and been brought together here. It is a good plan to de-brief yourself here after a visit to the real thing. Do not go to the museum first for the very simple reason that whilst it has authentic and splendid *objects d'art* from the Aescalapian, it lacks that veiled and enigmatic quality which pervades the open ruins and which has done so for 2500 years. For it is in this feeling that the real Epidaurus lies and not in its gathered weather-worn and posturing statues.

PERGAMON – THE TEMPLE

SO MUCH for Epidaurus in its splendour and its ignominy. It reached its peak from 370BC to 250BC when it was a place of major pilgrimage. In the second century AD it underwent renovations to try and compete with the new emerging force of Christianity. But the halcyon days were over and even the most bigoted devotee must have known its sun was on the wane.

It struggled on until AD426 when Emperor Theodosius II, a Christian, had it closed, doubtless at the insistence of the local clergy on account of its pagan overtones. It fell into disrepair, a state of affairs hastened by local Christians who used some of its stones for buildings dedicated to the glory of another god. To add insult to injury, in the seventeenth century AD a violent earthquake destroyed what had not already been vandalised. It may have been regarded then as a divine and just retribution for many hundreds years of past thaumaturgics but it could not destroy that aura of serenity which pervades it to this day.

Serene and calm Epidaurus may be, but because of the completeness of its destruction you may have difficulty getting in touch with the actual life and times of the Ancient Greek patient who visited it. The same cannot be said of the second great Temple of Aescalapius of the old world – Pergamon. For here, whilst a ruin, neither the forces of nature nor religious zeal have made it difficult to recognise a place of healing. By felicitous chance the surviving buildings, roads, fountains and the like give even the least creative twentieth century visitor a chance to give his jaded imagination fertile scope.

But first, what was it like at its peak? Pergamon is situated in the Western area of Anatolia, Turkey, which in the days of its glory was part of the Greek Empire. The name Pergamon has several meanings – castle, massive, fortress. Nowadays its modern counterpart is the town of Bergama. In the third century BC Alexander the Great paid it a visit, which must have created a certain chilliness in the population. It possessed a library of immense and famed proportion and which is said to have been given by Mark Antony to Cleopatra for their bijou and distant love nest. The volumes actually went to the town of Alexandria eventually to be destroyed by two extraordinary acts of pietistic vandalism which were to set back the then civilized world's knowledge of medicine and other scientific data several centuries. Everyone can help share the blame because the Christians burnt much of it in AD391 and the Moslems finished it off in AD642. The knowledge which books contain allows people to think, and that can be very dangerous. As we shall see later, the alleged romantic origins of the transfer are almost certainly wrong.

The ancient city itself, or acropolis, is set astride a hill which commanded views of all approaches, a standard position for this era. At its most populous it housed about 200 000 people. Much of its architectural splendour is now displayed in East Berlin at the Pergamon Museum. But it was not this fortified and brooding city which housed the Temple of Aescalapius. That was at the bottom of the hill, three kilometres or so from the main commercial centre, and, like Epidaurus, away from the hugger mugger of day to day existence. City and sanctuary were connected by the so called Holy Road.

The Temple was built about the fourth century BC by a local man called Archais. Apparently, he was hunting near Epidaurus, broke a bone in his foot and was treated at that medical centre. It healed well and, as a service to his own city, he brought several Aescalapiads from Epidaurus to Pergamon to build an Aescalapian of their own which quickly gained a good reputation. One of the reasons for this was that it was malaria free; no good going to have your headache cured only to die of malaria. You might as well have stayed at home.

Unlike Epidaurus, the interest in the Temple lies in what remains rather than what it was like 2000 years ago. The area which the building occupied has a kind of Red Square vastness and grandeur to it and there is much more left to see than at other similar Temples. As a result it is far easier to understand the workings of the place.

Five hundred years after its establishment its most famous son studied there. This was Galen, born in the second century AD and eventually to be bracketed with Hippocrates as the premier doctor of his time. He wrote of an additional Temple being built while he was a student and, indeed, his father was one of the designers. He was late in the day for Aescalapian worship for already Christians had their eyes on the profane pile and its days were numbered. An earthquake eventually destroyed it and doubtless vengeance from a just God was mooted, but whatever the cause the remaining saw-bones called it a day and it was abandoned to the birds, the sun and future archeologists.

These latter came along in 1927 when a German team was nosing about in the area and stopped to relax under a tree. To their amazement a sheep emerged from a bush opposite where they were sitting to be followed by a whole flock, rather like rabbits out of a conjurer's hat. A hidden cave was found and excavation revealed the Temple's most remarkable feature – the Holy Basement, of which more anon.

Now Pergamon lacks the serenity of leafy Epidaurus. It is large, short on trees and windy. Rather than a timeless and unhurried calm, there is given off even now the air of a clinic, well organised in the business of healing. There is an order about the place where religion and therapy work closely together with purpose and economy. There are few birds, little greenery and a muted presence only of noisy insects. In their place are a number of well preserved and functional architectural masterpieces.

The Holy Road from the old city is still here, at least the last 300 to 400 metres are. Well worn flagstones, three chariots wide, are flanked by the easily discernible remains of shops, taverns,

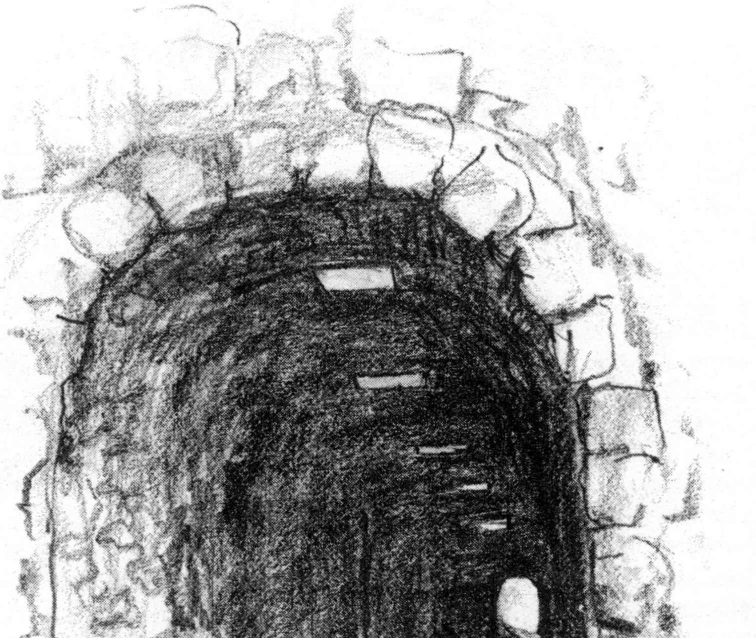

Holy Basement.
Pergamon

way-side shrines and the like. If you could not walk the distance from the city the Aescalapiads were not interested in you or your pathology. Obviously you were already too far gone and past their help. The priest doctors had a pragmatic view of life which at least kept their statistics looking good.

Today there is farmland between city and temple and you cannot walk the whole way from the lofty Acropolis. You have to approach the shrine by a circuitous route from Bergama through a Turkish army camp. It is somewhat ironic that the use of a camera or even stopping for a long look is forbidden as you approach one of the world's great monuments to the peaceful pursuit of caring.

You can walk along the last few remaining metres of the paved road, once having fought your way through the T-shirt sellers. Above the entrance used to be inscribed, 'By order of the Gods, here death does not roam'. Indeed, no records of death have survived. I rather fancy that when death was imminent those *in extremis* were whisked away to more secular surroundings. However, Aristeides, the Greek philosopher, had chronic ill health or so he claimed, and stayed for five years to enjoy the medical chit-chat and liturgical mysticism. He left us an invaluable legacy by giving details of the institution's protocol.

Galen, as we have seen, was the Temple's most famous Aescalapiad and he studied there from the age of seventeen until he was twenty-one. He later became medical officer to the school of gladiators which allowed him a pretty rapid turn-over of patients. He also wrote over 500 books on medicine, mainly anatomy, but they also gave us an insight into his philosophy. We shall look at him in some detail later.

But back to the Holy Road and so on into the sanctuary. To get there you go down three well worn steps from the road directly into a large reception or ceremony area. Once it was paved with gleaming white marble, but now it is gritty and pebbly, a base possibly made of 2000-year-old marble chips.

In the centre of this rectangular entrance is the much photographed stunted column on the surface of which is chiselled the likeness of several species of snake. Over the years it has become a kind of lodestone of medical practice. Whilst in its day it must have been a thing of reverence and beauty, now, standing there in splendid isolation, it merely displays a broken top and chipped base. It is said to have been carved in the time of Galen following on the observation of a man drinking from a cup of water into which two snakes had spat. Instead of dying as interested bystanders had supposed, the patient made a miraculous recovery from his illness. He drank in the first place because on presenting himself in this very ante-room he had been considered too ill to treat, so attempted suicide by this unusual method. Anyway, the seeming miracle gained his entry, the plaudits of the locals and confirmation of a therapeutic theory that Galen claimed to have had all along but uncharacteristically had been too reluctant to follow up on account of possibly fatal results. It also afforded confirmation of snakes being doctors' little helpers.

Having been passed as fit enough for treatment, the supplicant would have descended more steps into the propylaeum or entrance proper to the temple. So shall we.

Looking to the right there is seen to be a large open space encompassed by low walls. It is so undistinguished that if not carefully sought it would be missed, which would be a pity, for it used to house the library. It was the literary riches from here which went to Alexandria and were subsequently destroyed. The library originally had a high statue of Hadrianus adjacent to the entrance. It is still in existence and lodged in the Bergama museum.

In front of the propylaeum opens up the spacious and grand body of the Aescalapian proper. It is 130 metres long and 80 metres wide and now comprises a vast expanse of weeds, tumbled pediments, broken columns, marble building blocks and other detritus of a millennium of disinterest and desecration. At least, at first glance it appears to be that way, but in about the centre is a grotto-like structure into which a spring gurgles to fill a cool, limpid pool. As you would imagine, the waters are said to have healing properties; at least they taste cool and refreshing and are not obviously teeming with salmonella.

In actual fact this central area has always been open to be used as a ceremonial precinct. Its northern boundary is looked over by some ancient architectural grandeur for here, set against the length of the vast square, is a colonnade of Ionic columns. They run in splendid sentinel fashion 130 metres from the library to the theatre. Many are still complete despite having been erected in AD151 and partly damaged by an earthquake in AD175. They are massive, stark and quite magnificent.

They lead the eye to the open theatre, which is smaller than that at Epidaurus, but even so could cater for the artistic propensities of 3500 people at any one time.

While standing in the middle of the central concourse turn away from the colonnade and you will see the entrance to the basement or subterranean corridor spotted by chance in 1927. This and the building at its other end are the most exciting of the complex for right there, beautifully preserved and restored, is the Holy Basement along which the sick used to make their way to the sleeping area or abaton. It is 82 metres long, 2 metres wide and 2.7 metres high, paved and substantially built of the local stone and with holes set in the roof at regular intervals. It is solid enough to last another 2000 years if not for ever.

Those seeking cures watched some religious ceremony in the central open ground, cleansed themselves in the holy fountain to encourage pure thoughts and then made their way slowly down this unique corridor. As they did so the priests were above, crouching by the skylights, talking in stage whispers and giving suggestions for treatment and self-management to the sick and maimed below.

Today the restored gallery is in good shape, marble paved, cool and somewhat ill-lit from the roof squints. The patients have gone and, despite the gloom, so have the ghosts. What is left are latter-day visitors rude with health and who, apart from the noise of their quietly echoing foot steps, pass through in silence. They emerge blinking into the daylight to find themselves at the entrance to the Aescalapian's most remarkable and well preserved building, the dormitory or Temple of Telesphor.

PERGAMON – THE CURE

IN ITS time the sleeping place was two storeys high and outside steps are still to be seen. The upper storey comprised six adjoining sleeping chambers and the lower existing building is decorated with inset arches to produce a solid circular building. For the sick it was the holy of holies, for if a cure were to take place at all, this was the spot where it would happen.

The order of events was well laid down and practised over many years until it became almost an art form. Having traversed the basement in semi-darkness whilst listening to dismembered voices giving symbolic-type advice, the poor patient stumbled blinking into the daylight, doubtless in quite a state of psychic awareness. He or she then was wrapped in the skin of a sacrificial animal, a consciousness-raising if somewhat smelly arrangement. The abaton was entered, the already dim lights extinguished and sleep encouraged. There were very few windows in the circular room and the supplicants were ranged around the outside wall facing inwards. Looking at the surviving lower level now, it must have been able to cater for at least 100 at any one time.

The idea was that, having had treatment suggested whilst in transit, a cure would be dreamed up during the sleep. I have no doubt the induced and highly developed nervous state now apparent would at least stimulate some dreams, if only nightmares.

If this excitement was all too much and sleep was not forthcoming, the Aescalapiads were not above administering a little of the opium poppy. I suppose there was a limit to the length of time you could hang about until your charges sank into the arms of Morphus.

During the sleep, as we saw at Epidaurus, the god of Healing himself put in an appearance. As you would imagine with such credentials and such a build-up, he knew instinctively what to do – surgery, laying on of hands, touching the eyes of the blind and so on. If any treatment was prescribed it came in the form of herbs, baths, so-called mental training with modification of attitudes, swimming and walking. All sounds pretty sensible and modern but, in fact, these were the regular contemporary treatments and were expected by the invalids who had been conditioned by previous reports, wall inscriptions left by departed satisfied patients as well as priestly suggestions.

The vision, or, for the more cynical, the visual hallucination, then faded and a deep sleep followed during which part two of the cure took place. For it was during that log-like state when the holy animals of the shrine put in an appearance and licked the diseased part. Snakes, as we have seen, were the popular favourites, but dogs were also used.

In the National Museum in Athens is displayed a stone relief depicting Aescalapius treating someone's shoulder. In the background is the patient lying asleep on a couch with a snake licking the offending sore area. So the one sculpture depicts the sufferer dreaming of recovery and the deity rendering assistance. Shoulders and such like may be acceptable but I am not sure that the whole *mélange* has not got phallic overtones and I wonder if the sect did not have an erotic base. If it cured, as undoubtedly it often did, then I do not suppose it matters too much.

On awakening, the sleeper would whisper the advised therapy to the hovering duty Aescalapiad who doubtless would sagely nod, for who were they to question the deity, and he would administer accordingly. If, on waking, the poor patient had forgotten the name of the drug, he or she would be assured that forgiveness had not been forthcoming yet, more sedation would be given and sleep resumed. The fact that some people

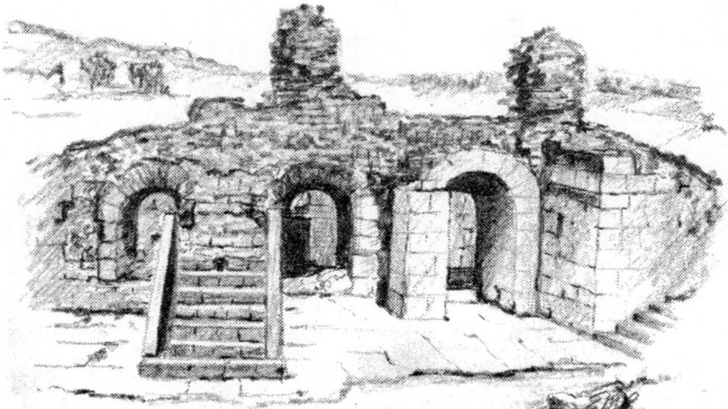

Temple of Telesphor or Abaton Pergamon.

stayed for years shows either that the administration of the sedation rather than the cure itself was the desired end, or that therapeutic success was as fickle and elusive then as it is now. There were spectacular recorded cures, however, and the Temple stonemasons were not reluctant to record them for posterity. Failures are notable by their absence, a human foible which indicates that the more things change, the more they are the same.

Epidaurus had more engraved recordings than Pergamon, so let us look at a few from these two great centres of healing.

Ambrosia of Athens came being blind in one eye. Apparently she was sceptical but went through the process. Sure enough Aescalapius appeared and promised a cure if she would give a silver pig as her memorial. She agreed, so he cut out the eye, poured in some drug, replaced the organ and she woke up cured. Sounds both effective and gruesome.

A boy had lost his voice. After the usual ritual a thanks offering was requested within a year and to the surprise of his father the boy piped up 'I promise that'. They were his first words for months.

Euhippus turned up with a spear point fixed in his jaw; sounds nasty. During the incubation Aescalapius pulled it out, and the following morning the old soldier walked out with it in his hand. I bet he dined out on that story for years.

Tales are recorded of crutches being thrown out, paralysis licked away, hearing restored and the like. One mother had a daughter swollen with dropsy. The girl remained at home while the mother slept in the Temple. There she dreamed that her daughter had had her head cut off by Aescalapius, then she was hung upside down and all the water drained out and the head fitted back. When the woman returned home sure enough she found the girl in good health, if a trifle shaken.

Pregnancy and sexual problems feature frequently and Cleo tells how she had been pregnant for five years but had not been able to come into labour. After the appropriate incubation she immediately left the precinct (remember nobody can die, or be born in the Temple) and was promptly delivered of a boy who got up and washed himself in a nearby fountain. How she explained that one away to her mother is tantalisingly omitted.

I suppose many of the patients had what we would now call a psychosomatic condition and some hysterical conversion. Feeling they were in contact with a divine power who embraced their problems, the symptoms had subsided. It certainly won glory for the god of Healing. The scribes were in the pay of the Temple and so would only be inclined to record success; the era of the double blind trial was some thousands of years in the future.

Those who did benefit were not ungrateful, and have left for us mute testimony of their spectacular cures. As well as a gift on entry, a mark of thanks was demanded on departure and there exist today many examples of these so-called votives. They usually took the form of a terracotta or marble or even gold representation of the part of the anatomy which had been successfully treated. The biggest collection appears to be in the museum at Corinth. It is housed in a special and usually locked room, but is worth seeking out. One wall is hung about with models of breasts, genitalia, arms, hands, hind quarters, uteri, bowels and brains all of which have been locally excavated. Many are of childrens' anatomical parts. The most exquisite example is in the museum at Bergama close to Pergamon. It is a solid gold representation of an ear.

The standard of craftsmanship varies from the crude and primitive to genuine works of art but there can be no doubt that all were offered to Aescalapius in the heart-felt desire to give thanks for the healing he had brought about.

Well, eventually the party was over and the devotee left the Temple of Telesphor and emerged with glory in the soul if not yet fully sound in wind and limb. Between the incubation area and the ceremonial area at the entrance is the most holy place of Aescalapion – the Temple of Aescalapius itself. It is strategically placed and had to be passed by everyone on their way out. Here the votives or donations were extracted, their size or splendour depending on the finances or place in society of the patient.

The Temple itself is still there, circular, solid and retaining the roof's supporting columns. The roof has gone and if in times past it was the holy of holies for the priests, if not the visitors, today it lacks the design, majesty and fascination which characterise many other parts of this complex.

The healing Temple at Pergamon was the most famous of its kind in the ancient world, attracting supplicants from far and wide to what was, I suppose, a huge clinic, almost a city conurbation. Not only failing health was catered for, but advice was sought and given by the god on matters of business, marriage, and politics. Such seeming universal wisdom doubtless gave the physician priests ideas above their station, and that imagined omnipotence must have contributed to their eventual downfall. But they delivered the goods to a large enough group of believers not only to survive, but in their time to grow into a big business, with appropriate financial rewards.

Because of its immense size and fine state of preservation as well as its well-recorded historical reputation, Pergamon cannot fail to impress. Yet it lacks the tranquillity and restfulness of Epidaurus, being windy, treeless and exposed to the merciless Mediterranean sun. In the twentieth century, carrying out the contemplative art which was supposed to be the corner-stone of the institution's medical prowess is difficult to imagine. But therapeutic success it had and that is, I suppose, the yardstick by which to measure its existence.

THE ISLAND OF COS

IF THERE is any snippet of ancient medical history that a dweller in the twentieth century would admit to knowing, it is the fact that Hippocrates is regarded as the Father of Medicine and, maybe, that he lived on the Aegean island of Cos. This must be true because the city fathers of the present-day metropolis of Cos, as well as those on the island proper, have seen fit to clearly mark and encourage a visit to a couple of monuments associated with Hippocrates and medicine. For it is here on this small island just off the Turkish coast there exists the plane tree under which the venerable old gentleman is said to have taught his students.

Now, let's not go overboard about this. There is no doubt about there being a tree, but as the life span of plane trees is only 400 to 500 years and the old boy lived 2500 years ago, then a fair discrepancy is manifest, one which is far beyond that allowed by poetic licence. In fairness, the local guide books do say it is an offshoot of the original and attempt to salvage some local pride by claiming it to be the oldest tree in Europe. It would be charitable to allow them that.

In any event, as I say, a gnarled and bent old tree does exist not, as you may imagine, as part of a leafy arbour close to a serpent-entwined shrine, but very near to the city centre itself. It almost fills a tiny square behind the island's Administration House.

As befits its great age, it is bowed, twisted and hollowed and supported on all sides by tubular steel scaffolding. It is protected all round by a wall topped by railings up to two metres tall, but its leafy branches are not confined by such man-made obstacles and hang over the fender. A couple of small benches allow the starry-eyed visitor to sit and indulge in whatever reverie he can – not so easy when the tree is hemmed in by a mosque, a couple of restaurants and several shops all seemingly designed to encroach noisily on any quiet contemplation. Strangely, the only plaque adjacent to the tree tells not of its connection with Hippocrates but of building the mosque.

Having marvelled at the tree, you can then turn to the other medical feature of Cos, its Aescalapian, for, with Epidaurus and Pergamon, this makes up the third leg of the great triumvirate of Temples of Healing of ancient times. Each has different characteristics and the temple on Cos has the most grandiose setting. This is all to the good as it is the most popular amongst those keen on following the healing trail. If only one is to be visited, this one will generate most wonderment.

From about the fifth century BC the cult spread from Epidaurus to Corinth, to Athens in 420 BC, Pergamon, Delphi and finally Cos. In fact, the edifice was not built until after the death of Hippocrates, so whilst there was a medical tradition on the island, the great man himself did not learn his medicine at the Temple. This was built on a spot chosen with great care to fit the environmental criteria for such places: quiet surroundings, preferably malaria-free, a good climate and fresh running water for cleansing purposes. An altar was erected in a cypress grove, still identifiable, in the middle of the fourth century BC. This was followed by a small temple built around a spring, again a physical feature still in existence. In the second century a richer temple and colonnade were added and works of art installed.

The cult thrived and a Pan Hellenic festival was held every four years. Such affairs of sport and art always attracted crowds and – then as now – were a source of publicity and revenue. The resulting cash flow allowed more colonnades to be added and the Temple was enlarged by being tiered up a hill. There is no doubt but that the emigrant divines had as big a success in the temporal world of finance and building as in the therapeutic field of healing, for the sanctuary they established survived for centuries. Their entrepreneurial skills manifested themselves by the building of edifices for worship and accommodation, whereas the teacher in the old school under the tree had no oratory and made you find your own lodgings. The original master craftsman concluded that the tabernacle he built was in men's hearts and not in bricks and mortar. But there was a subtle difference between the Aescalapiads who set up shop, so to speak, on Cos and those who were affiliated with Epidaurus and Pergamon, for on Cos they were not priests but trained physicians who worshipped Aescalapius, their medical expertise taking precedence over their religious duties and not the other way round.

The site of the Temple on Cos is still there, of course, and presents now as a shady, quiet and relaxing sanctuary being located about four kilometres outside the township and its famous plane tree. It is approached in the last 300 metres or so by a gentle curving road which runs through a triple row of scented cedars of Lebanon. Suddenly you emerge from this overhung way into a sunlit car park, and right there, massively raised before you, is the most spectacularly landscaped Temple. It is tiered into three levels of impressively large platforms separated from each other by terraced walls and connected by broad flights of marble stairs. The majesty of Epidaurus is evident, but it has been enhanced by the order that has been given to the partially restored ruins. It is set in woodland surrounds like Epidaurus, but lacks the size and easily recognisable old buildings of Pergamon. But the builders' use of the natural features of the site make up for any deficiencies. It is hardly credible that it is about 2400 years old.

An external stairway of twenty-four steps leads from what is now the carpark to the first layer or andiron. Away to the left and at the edge of a flat, pebbly parade-ground-like area are the foundations of rooms. This first level was said to contain the School of Anatomy and Pathology and these chambers were used by patients either for sleeping or consultation. They are of passing interest and along with the odd statue plinth should not divert you from crunching your way across the open area towards the embankment wall built into the hillside. This structure extends along the whole length of the expanse and is colonnaded. In the niches of the colonnade were statues, probably representing deities. Apart from one, all are now empty. The exception lies just to the left of the next staircase and is a likeness of the god Pan, holding a flute and with water running from beneath his feet. The water flows into a large stone ornamental pond before the marble statue and eventually overflows into the andiron itself to produce a muddy area in which young visitors can get thoroughly dirty. Doubtless it is a perpetual spring and has flowed from ancient times.

Away to the left outside the perimeters are the ruins of stone villas probably of a secular nature although a number of votives were found there. The whole platform is about as cluttered as a football field on a Monday morning, and about the same size.

Thirty well maintained steps lead to the second level. At the top you come immediately upon the most ancient structure of the Temple, the altar to Aescalapius himself. Little remains – a rectangle of stone, ill-placed and incomplete – but it lies at the centre of the whole complex. To one side of the altar are the ruins of the small Temple to Aescalapius dating from the third century BC. As at Epidaurus, it may be that the altar lay just at the entrance to the Temple, a structure now only identifiable by two propped-up Ionic columns.

To the east on the other side of the altar is the most photographed area of the Aescalapian – the Temple of Apollo, father of Aescalapius. Seven fine Corinthian columns exist and partly outline the rectangular holy spot. Annually on this site a reconstructive tableau depicting a reaffirmation of the Hippocratic Oath is enacted by men dressed as priests and women fitted out in long white robes more reminiscent of vestal virgins than early doctors. Perhaps they are token patients. Nevertheless, because of the form and shape of the restored columns this is the spot where it is easiest to appreciate the historical ambience and feel that here one is at the very centre of the ancient art of healing.

Away to the west, past the rather crude pair of early Ionic columns, past the trough covered with a marble slab and which used to act as the Treasury, past the ruin of another small temple dedicated to Nero, are the remains of a staircase which leads to the surrounding woods. The trees were there from earliest times, the forebears of these giants, of course. This is the so-called hallowed forest within the enclosure of which again nobody was allowed to be born or to die. They were pretty keen on this at that time and it was a rule sometimes extended to whole areas, Delos island, for instance. This even though Apollo and Artemis were born there. Anyway, the forest now is studded with tall trees which look pretty forbidding when viewed from the sunlit safety of the Temple. It appears to be the last place anyone would want to give birth.

From the centre of the second level are more marble steps, sixty this time, leading to the third andiron. There are 114 steps in all from the bottom to the most holy area of the complex, the great Temple of Aescalapius of Cos. The temple dates from the second century BC, was built in the Doric style and measures thirty-four metres by eighteen metres. It is a complete ruin now and only from the surviving parapet wall can be seen the footings of the 104 columns it boasted in its hey-day. It contained great statues of Aescalapius and Hygieia. Around the periphery of this andiron are the foundations of many small rooms used during the incubation period of treatment.

On the eastern side of the ruin is a short column surmounted by a marble slab. Its overhang is ideal for sitting under to get away

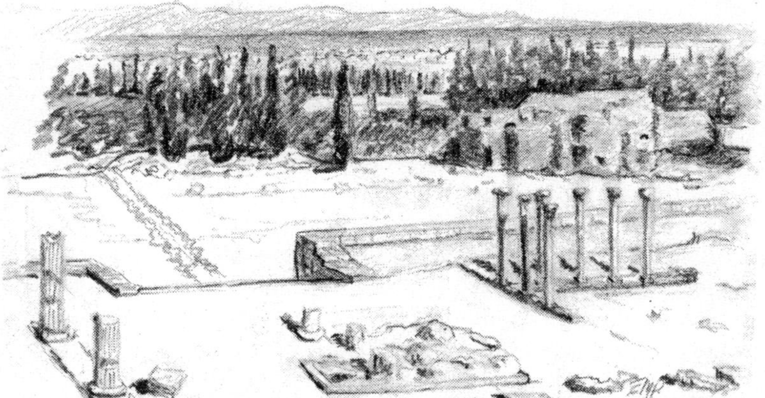

Aescalapian Sanctuary – Cos

from the Mediterranean sun and to eat your sandwiches whilst contemplating the view. Doubtless it was an altar in its time and is inscribed ICXP so was probably Christian. Even Christians have to eat.

Having reached the pinnacle of the Aescalapian, now is the time to turn and look north, back over the terraces and the entrance, back over the sweeping approach, onto the town of Cos, white and ochre in the distance, over the cobalt-blue Aegean to the distant hills of mainland Turkey. Not only is it a breath-taking view but, apart from the ubiquitous cicadas and the faint distant rustling of the trees, all is silence. More than that, the instant is made even more emotive by remembering that this scene was looked down upon by the devotees of the god of Healing for over 1000 years.

I have outlined the function of the Temples of Healing of Aescalapius. They held sway for many hundreds of years as a form of treatment, a cure and a source of comfort to countless thousands of ordinary men and women. They were mystical, spiritual yet pagan institutions. They gloried in a god who was, at best, a benign father image dispensing harmless advice to a gullible population and at worst, a false bolster to a distressed and ill humanity. The visible legacies he caused to be left are massive and beautiful monuments to the false premise that man can attain immortality. As the chill wind moans through the remaining Doric columns and grass grows among the footings, we look on the faded glory and remember that all man-made objects are liable to decay.

Two new ideas eroded the power of Aescalapius, the advent of Christianity with its promise of redemption and the love of its deity, and, second, the emergence of a new medical thinking. This latter grew for many years in tandem with the old order, but eventually was to survive it, greatly modified, it is true, but still recognisable today. For as the mysteries of Aescalapius faltered and decayed, the pragmatism of Hippocrates and Galen hung on into fairly modern times.

But the old order is still remembered with some affection. Its birth place around the Aegean is still visited and its methods are still cause for wonder.

The isles of Greece, the isles of Greece!
Where Sappho loved and sung,
Where grew the arts of war and peace
Where Delos rose and Phoebus sprung!
Eternal summer gilds them yet,
But all, except their sun, is set.

(BYRON *Don Juan*)

HIPPOCRATES – HIS LIFE AND TIMES

I SUPPOSE Hippocrates (460-370 BC) is the best known single name in medical history. What he meant to the Greeks who came after him, to the people of the Middle Ages or Renaissance or, indeed, what he means today, is all the same, namely, that by a convoluted historical process he has become the embodiment of the ideal physician. He is seen now as he was then as being wise, knowledgeable, unruffled, caring, avuncular rather than paternal and the originator of a code of behaviour which has survived some thousands of years. In short, he is seen as the Father of European medicine.

Probably because of this ancient mystique he has been burdened with the fiction of having written, alone and unaided, all those catchy aphorisms which bear his name. It is extremely doubtful whether he tossed off more than a few – others probably added to them over the years.

That he was small of stature, that he travelled widely and that he died in Larissa in the eastern part of the Greek mainland is about the extent of our certain knowledge. The rest is conjecture. But really, except for pedantic historians, it does not matter too much, for it is as convenient to collect wise principles from 2000 years ago under one name as it is to heap abuse onto a single unfortunate for telling of life's misfortunes, as happened to Cassandra.

Only two contemporary references to Hippocrates exist. One is in the Dialogues of Plato in which we learn that the Aescalapiad Hippocrates was a native of Cos, taught students for money and was well-known about the other centres of healing in the Eastern Mediterranean. From the other reference, attributed to the physician and historian Ctesias, it is apparent that the old boy devised a kind of home-spun philosophy regarding medical practice and that the resulting folksy pearls were used to attract medical aspirants from distant parts. It is probably not true that he brought together followers of Aescalapius, for the Temple to that god, as we have seen, was not established on Cos until after the days of Hippocrates when it was set up as some form of opposition, or at least as a co-belligerant. They probably managed to keep each other honest.

Four biographies do exist, but were written long after his death and seem more to idealise the man than to set down a true history. They do have some common ground, however. For instance, each concludes that he became an itinerant healer for some years because, believe it or not, he was reputed to have burned down a medical library and so had to flee the island. One writer places this act of academic vandalism at the rival establishment of Cnidus, on the mainland across from Cos. Another authority put it on Cos itself. What price the avuncular and caring image now? At least it made him human, although burning down a library is going a bit far.

At all events, one of the biographies, that by Soranus of Ephesus, purports to give us some background. His father was said to have been the physician Heraclides, a man who could trace his ancestory back to Hercules and Aescalapius himself, no less. Hippocrates was born in the first year of the eighteenth Olympiad, which puts the date at 460 or 459 BC. He was taught medicine by his father, sophistry by Gorgeus and philosophy by Democritus.

When the doubtless precocious child considered himself competent in medical skills he left Cos and travelled all over

Greece. According to Soranus he gained there a reputation for being a very skilled practitioner, so much so that the then King of Macedonia engaged him to treat his tuberculosis. The nature of the regal symptoms has been lost, but as resolution of this condition defied all therapeutic efforts until the mid-twentieth century, the task must have been awesome. The Master was not abashed, however, said something along the lines that it was all in the mind, and, so it is said, promptly effected a cure. Despite the historian's certainty, it all seems too good to be true and probably has lost something in the translation.

Later Hippocrates was invited by the Illyrians to cast out the plague then decimating their country. Now, at the time Illyuria was at war with the Greeks and, being a Greek, Hippocrates felt it improper to treat the opposition. He realised, however, that the disease could spread to his own side so repaired to Attica to await events. For similar patriotic reasons he refused a call to go to the Persian court of Artaxerxes, despite the fat fee offered. He seems to have been a Greek first and a physician second.

This somewhat unusual selflessness in a medical man prompted the Athenians to give him an illuminated address. In it they allowed him to be initiated into the 'great mysteries'. Naturally, being mysteries these were unspecified but as it was all to be at government expense he accepted. The outcome is still unclear, and anyway has now lost all meaning.

About the same time the Athenians crowned him during a gymnastic contest with a wreath of gold valued at a thousand gold coins. The city state continued to go overboard with Hippocrates for, in recognition of the fact that Cos produced such a public-spirited and knowledgeable son, they also granted to Coan children equal rights with the children of Athens. Finally, to cap it off, they gave this paragon Athenian citizenship and a life-long annuity.

He seems to have become a legend in his own lifetime which may have all seemed a very satisfactory arrangement for Hippocrates but, regrettably, we have no proof that it was not all a figment of the biographer's imagination.

Neverthelesss, Hippocrates did exist. He was revered throughout Greece and died at the age of ninety in the province of Thessaly, appropriately enough, near the alleged birthplace of Aescalapius

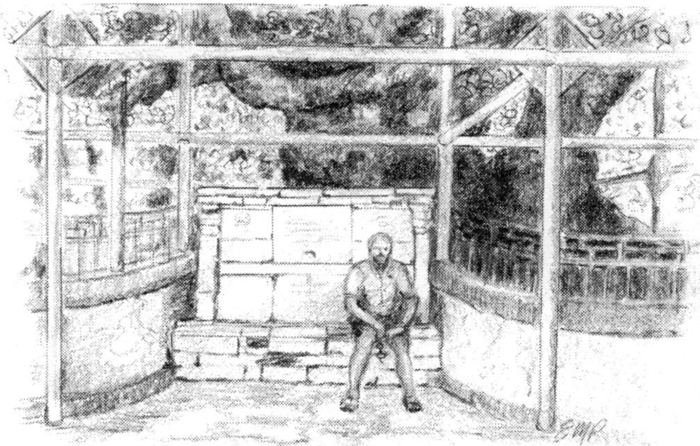

Sitting under Hippocrates Tree. — Cos

himself. A beehive was set upon the tomb at Larissa and the honey it produced was said, as you may well imagine, to have had great curative powers.

Unlike Socrates, Pericles, Sophocles and others, we do not know what Hippocrates looked like. The other great men lived in Athens and the master sculptors of the day moulded their likenesses for posterity but there is no known, authentic statue of the old doctor. The government of Cos eventually issued coins bearing the physician's portrait and four of these are still in existence. The snag is that they were struck 800 years after his death, although the features possibly could be based on an early painting since lost. What is shown is a bald, thick-set man, forehead wrinkled with care and concern, or maybe taxation problems, and a rather wavy, well-trimmed beard. It could be anyone, really, but he does have the face of a man with whom you could entrust your abdominal pain, ear ache or pregnancy.

In any event, as time has gone on the supposed medical virtues of Hippocrates have made him appear larger than life. This is partly due to his dedicated career but more to his purported writings, the so-called *Corpus Hippocraticum*.

It has long been accepted that this collection of ancient *bon mots* is not the work of one man but probably represents the accumulated medical literature of the period. The books date from the third and fourth century BC and about sixty are recognised as making up the set. The earliest surviving manuscript is from the tenth century AD. As these dates of production and printing are a considerable distance apart, their validity must be in dispute. In the end, any mediaeval monastic herbalist could have added his favourite poultice recipe, and we would be none the wiser.

The original efforts were assembled in the great library at Alexandria which was established by Ptolemy when he was granted Egypt in the carve-up after the death of Alexander the Great. Over a period of four hundred years this library accumulated what the far-seeing founders no doubt hoped would be the sum total of human knowledge at the time. It eventually held 700 000 books and possessed a unique reputation for scholastic endeavour. The incumbent librarians sought out the writings of Hippocrates and other Aegean medical authors to keep faith with the original vision. The whole lot was catalogued under the master's name which, on contemplation, is somewhat curious in view of Hippocrates's alleged propensity to ignite book collections.

Having housed all this wealth of knowledge, the library's subsequent destruction by fire hardly bears contemplation. The accumulated wisdom contained in books commonly brings about new ideas, a questioning of the old order and maybe a general desire for change. In other words, inflammatory notions to an Ogygian devotee of the status quo. So perhaps we should be surprised not that the sublime establishment was razed, but that it took these zealots so long to get round to it.

If the story of the life of Hippocrates is sketchy, the writings of his *Corpus* do survive, however tenuous the connection, and deserve a chapter of their own.

HIPPOCRATES – HIS WRITINGS

AS WE have seen, the writings attributed to the master physician, Hippocrates, are much more likely to have been the result of the fertile outpourings of many medical experts over a large number of years. They were collected under the general heading of *Corpus Hippocraticum*. Within this massive work the contents were divided into several sections.

The Oath is, of course, the best-known piece of succint writing attributed to the old master. In fact, it is thought to antedate Hippocrates and to have been added to the collection later during its compilation. The reason given for including these as second thoughts is its allusion to prohibiting abortion and contraception. These strictures fitted more easily into the tenets of the later Christian Church than did the more freewheeling ideas of earlier times. Oddly enough, in other of his attributed writings, Hippocrates frequently refers to active methods of procuring an abortion with the use of pessaries. But, all in all, the code of medical conduct, purity and care which the Oath lays down embodies the kind of attitudes which any civilised culture would like to ascribe to its favourite father-like physician. Regrettably, they seem to be honoured more in the breach than the observance.

The second most famous set of his writings are the Aphorisms, among the most cherished of which are:

- Life is short and the Art long; Opportunity fleeting; Experience dangerous; Judgment difficult.
- For extreme diseases extreme strictness of treatment is most efficacious.
- When sleep puts an end to delirium it is a good sign.
- Those diseases that medicine does not cure are cured by the knife. Those that the knife does not cure are cured by fire. Those that fire does not cure must be considered incurable.

And so on and so on and so on. There are several hundred of these homilies altogether, and they all have a folksy ring about them, a homespun philosophy. I suppose that if the only treatment at your disposal is pretty empirical, then you inevitably learn to observe the progress of illness to its natural end, which was often fatal. The doctors of old also studied people as a whole, in their own environment. Laboratory tests were many centuries away.

Hippocrates, it is said, wrote a book entitled *The Sacred Disease*. Strangely enough it is not clear even now which disease was being described, but it was most probably epilepsy. In it he, or whoever the real author was, attacks the superstitions which surrounded the condition, together with those who trade on its frightening features, or the 'magicians, purifiers, charletons and quacks' as he calls them. These faith-healers regarded epilepsy as a divine illness and forbade the eating of certain foods such as fish or fowl on the grounds that they were impure and their consumption showed impiety. Hippocrates would have none of this gibberish, adding it was the grotesque contortions of the sufferer during an attack which gave the bogus appearance of supernatural visitation. So far so good, but then the writer lets us down by asserting that the fits are brought on by the effects of wind and rain on a susceptible constitution.

The treatise on anatomy in the Hippocratic collection is short on detail. The reason is simple – the Greeks did not dissect human bodies. First, it was forbidden on religious grounds and, second, their respect for the dead was greater than their curiosity about them. The text did manage to get the skeleton pretty right, presumably from chanced-upon remains. Knowledge of blood circulation did not exist and the differences between arteries and veins was not understood, despite the fact that a previous civilisation had shown it in some detail, as we have seen. Nerves were confused with ligaments and described as ending nowhere.

Descriptions of the heart were probably made by a later writer for a fair degree of accuracy is shown. The chambers of the organ are described as being rough, as though eaten away, the left more so than the right. This, so it was claimed, was because the left contains a greater amount of air and heat. The upper chambers of the heart, or auricles, were said to be bellows which blew air into the lower segment, or ventricles. This mechanism was written up as 'the work of a cunning artificer'.

Because so little internal examination took place, speculation was rife as to the functioning of the body, especially the passage of fluid and gases. Hence arose the theory of the 'humours' and of the 'pneumas'. The humours determined men's or women's constitutions or temperaments as well as their health. The pneumas and their movement accounted for consciousness. The humours were listed as blood, phlegm, yellow bile and black bile. Black bile was probably the changed and blackened blood which appears in vomit and faeces after bleeding in the gut and is of serious import. The other humours were regarded as permanent constituents of normal blood that changed with the onset of disease to become pathological. The sacred disease of epilepsy, for instance, was said by some authorities to be due to an excess of phlegm in the brain.

Vagaries of the weather and their effect on the body had a lengthy write-up, which is more than can be said for the modern textbook. Weather was thought to have a significant effect on the humours. City dwellers exposed to hot winds and heads full of phlegm, were poor eaters and suffered from indigestion. Cities open to the northerly cold winds were peopled by inhabitants who were said to be bilious, thin, constipated but who at least had clear heads. It's an ill wind et cetera. I wonder if any long term follow-up has been done on this rather acute observation?

A book on the epidermis listed changes of weather as being very important in the waxing and waning of skin diseases, and noted that different medicines were needed for different seasons.

Case histories abound which tell of maladies associated with movement of the bile, blood and any other body fluids. Spring sees blood rising like the sap to cause dysentery, nose bleeds and, perhaps, allergy. As summer progresses, blood gives way to yellow bile. Autumn is hostile to nature, it is claimed, and the yellow bile is gradually replaced by black bile and treatment modified accordingly. At the same time as all this is going on, the caring clinician has to bear in mind the temperament that those humours bring, namely, phlegmatic, sanguine, choleric and melancholic personalities.

The less well known theory of the pneumas, or vital air, was developed on Cos. Briefly, it postulates the passage of air through the blood vessels to cool the body. The air is then brought together in the lungs and breathed out.

Diseases of women and their anatomy and physiology have a treatise to themselves which makes strange reading now. Take the womb or uterus, for instance. It was said to be warmer on the left side and so produced male embryos which, on account of the heat, matured more quickly than the female. When fertilised, the embryo drew breath into itself in order to develop, it was said, a coating or crust 'like baked bread'. This crust retained a hole in the middle through which further breaths could be taken. From this hole the umbilical cord eventually developed. There was no menstruation during pregnancy because the mother's blood was drawn into the foetus to help nourish it. In the end the foetus brought on its own birth by increasing agitation when the food supply ran low, so breaking out of the surrounding membrane.

It all sounds so simple and cosy, almost Arcadian. Baking a pie, milking a cow, gathering in hay, producing a baby, they are all the same, artless and all part of the grand unfathomable design of life. Where did we go wrong?

Perhaps the area where the Hippocratic physicians excelled most was in clinical observation. Untrammelled by the trappings of modern medicine such as electronmicroscopy, floroscopy, computer printouts or even thermometers, observation was honed to an art form. The well known book of the *Corpus Hippocraticum* concerning observation was called *Prognostics*. It starts, reasonably enough, with the face. Features such as hollow eyes, sharp nose, cold ears, parched skin, high colour and so forth received detailed appraisal and the likely outcome was given for a sufferer of these appearances. It seems that if you start to sleep with the whites of the eye visible when formerly the lids have been closed, that is a deadly sign. So, too, is looseness or whitening of the lips. Innumerable signs and their hidden meanings are listed, from positions adopted whilst sleeping to where sweating occurs on the body; from the type of sediment found in the urine to the size of blisters.

Its companion volume is called *Epidemic*. This concerns itself more with the mode of life, manner of speaking, nature of thoughts and so forth. Altogether there are seven books of *Epidemic* and they contain many case histories which give enough detail for us to make a diagnosis of, among others, malaria, puerperal fever or septicaemia 2000 years on. Telling of tuberculosis is also common, and the thesis notes how the cough improves during the summer to return in autumn and be followed by more deaths in winter. The cause of this odd seasonal disease was, of course, a complete mystery to the ancients but treatment was well documented in the sensible areas of rest, warmth, different foods, sympathy and encouragement.

Preventive medicine was also practised in the form of exercise and the eating of various foods. Cereals were considered to be cooling and drying, meats heating and windy, beans astringent and flatulence-producing, peas laxative and so on. It has quite a modern feel, really.

As regards exercise, obese people should walk faster, bathing should be more frequent in summer and the lean should wash more than the fat. Emetics should be reserved for the winter and enemas for the summer. Either way, the latter should be of milk in lean people and salt water in the obese. The detail is mind-numbing, covering, as it does, virtually every mental attitude and physical condition of free men and slaves.

Just one example in detail should suffice. Barley gruel is listed as a food to sustain the invalid. So far so good. But pages are devoted to arguments about whether the gruel should be strained or unstrained; if strained, the type of cloth to use; whether, if unstrained, it should remain thus throughout the illness or just for the first six days or before or after the crisis; whether the barley should be freshly gathered or not. It all appears to be the medical

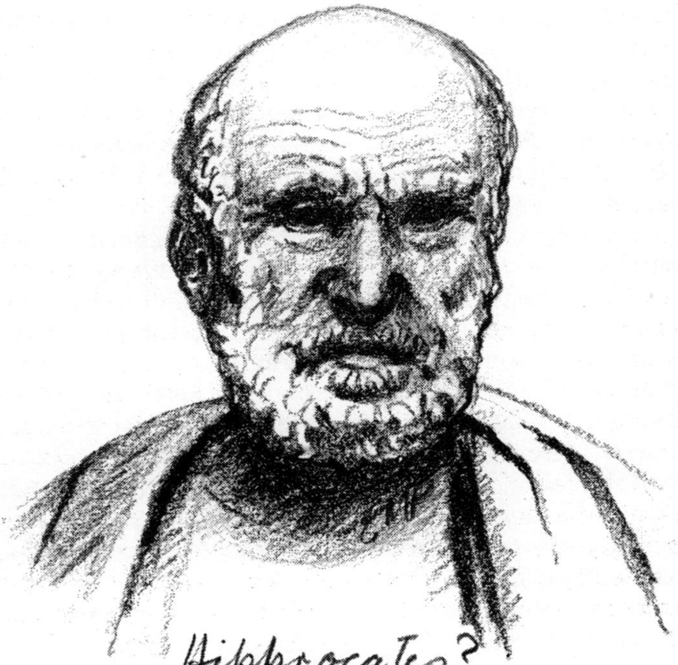

Hipprocates?
Marble bust in British Museum.

equivalent of the theological argument about how many angels can dance on the head of a pin.

Bathing gets a good write-up and at least it would have done no harm. But it was said it should be in a covered place and the soap should be warmed. I rather think that refers to liquid soap made of powder and olive oil. Sponges were to be used instead of a scraper. The use of the latter seems to indicate a bath was regarded as a luxury or a form of medication for such was the encrustation of grime that once a plunge was taken it had to be chipped away. Bathing, it was averred, suits pneumonia, but not looseness of the bowels or bleeding from the nose. I suppose some of these therapies survived into this century, until, in fact, antibiotics did away with such fussy nicities as warming the soap.

Intervention beyond foodstuffs, bathing and prayer was confined to bleeding, cautery, fomentations and the treatment of wounds and fractures. Fomentation relieved pain and comprised sitting in hot water in a bronze vessel with a sponge between patient and container. Bleeding was usually carried out on the arm by incising a vein at the elbow. If the condition it was supposed to cure was acute, then bleeding was carried on until the patient fainted. Cautery involved heating a metal rod which was then inserted through the skin to drain an abscess. Doubtless the apprentice held the patient down during the ghastly performance. It sounds pretty horrendous even for those days.

These were regarded as medical procedures and were carried out by a physician, but surgery proper was also undertaken. Not surgery in the sense of fossicking about in some steamy entrails to cobble up a hernia or shell out a gallbladder. No, Hippocratic surgery was more to do with bones and adjacent soft tissues. There are books entitled *Fractures* and *Joints* and both contain recommended treatments which have a modern flavour. This is perhaps not surprising as the setting of broken limbs should follow common-sensical pathways for it is a practical specialty whose exponents are purposeful operators not usually given to breast-beating over psychological nuances.

It states, for example, that if an arm is broken the fractured ends should be pressed into position using the manipulator's palms. When the limb is bound up the patient should have his hand placed lower than his elbow so that the blood may flow to the extremity. The bandage should run from below upwards and compression be applied to the break. When the swelling has subsided the bones will be found to be more mobile and ready for adjustment. A tubular splint of wooden slats can then be applied. Many other fracture treatments are listed, and whilst we know from recovered skeletons they were successful, I wonder how the patient stood the manipulations.

Instructions on the straightening of the spine are intriguing. The written warning that the manoeuvres are not recommended by the experts for use by the casual operator should alert us to their diabolical nature. Tuberculosis commonly deformed the spine and the popular layman's method of straightening it was as follows: The patient is to be bound to a ladder with feet pointing down if the deformity is high in the back, and upwards if low in the back. The ladder is then leaned against a wall on which an assistant is stood. The assistant then lifts the ladder vertically and lets it down smoothly and often so that it repeatedly strikes the ground. The object was to jolt the vertebrae into some semblance of true alignment.

That was the do-it-yourself method undertaken with the help of a friend and did not have the stamp of medical approval. The accepted method, however, was almost as grotesque, at least according to our lights. This involved lying the patient prone on a board by a wall. A plank, suitably padded, was then laid across the humped and tuberculous back and hinged at the other end to the wall. Incredibly, the free end was then pressed down onto the deformity using all the weight of the doctor's most muscular assistant. Again the success rate is tantalisingly not recorded, nor for that matter the opinions of the patients.

It is in the book *Fractures* that the so-called Hippocratic bench is described. This is a thing of straps, pulleys and windlasses used for straightening various bits of human anatomy. Dislocations were realigned with no more than a crack and a scream.

Living in an era when-hand-to-hand fighting was a way of life (or death), wounds, especially head wounds, were commonplace. Hence the doctors of the time became experts of trauma and tales of treatment are minutely detailed and splendid in their good sense. Imhotep would have been proud of them.

Finally, there were instructions for surgical operators – keep the nails short; practise with both hands; the thumb should be able to oppose each finger; and the whole *tour de force* should be done with ability, grace, speed, elegance, readiness and resourcefulness. It would seem a surgeon was to be bracketed, as regards facility and movement, with a musician or athlete. Doubtless some would have had the dexterity of an orang-utan playing a violin but at least they were well taught.

AFTER HIPPOCRATES

THE ISLAND of Cos was not, of course, the only centre of medical teaching and excellence. It is perhaps the most famous, partly because of Hippocrates and partly because of the romantically placed Temple of Aescalapius and the twisted old tree beloved of modern physicians. But other centres had their devotees and secret potions.

Across from Cos on the Turkish mainland was the school of Cnidos. It had a different outlook on medicine for its top staff members painstakingly classified symptoms as diseases and thereupon produced a remedy for each. For them diagnosis and treatment were the end-all and be-all of medicine, unlike their neighbours where observation of the patient as a whole took precedence. In the long run this latter *modus operandi* proved the more acceptable and survives to this day. The mainland faculty were not party to such fol-de-rols as teasing out the cause of disease or thinking through prognosis and all that philosophical stuff, so passed into comparative obscurity.

The school of Cnidos did produce some literature from its cloisters which has survived. It consists mainly, as we have seen, of long lists of symptoms each graced with the name of a disease. Hence there were seven diseases of the bile, twelve of the bladder, three types of phthisis and so on. It was a mind-numbing catalogue which, strangely, produced few remedies, merely an eminently forgettable faculty membership. Other medical tracts survive from Sicily and North Africa, but details are scant.

All these volumes represent the accumulated medical knowledge of the times. They were lodged in their early days in the library at Pergamon, the ruined shell of which, as we noted, still exists. Cos had a library but no structure has survived. After Hippocrates others felt compelled to record their experiences and many were stored away. All were written in the Ionic dialect which thus became the language of Greek science, somewhat as Latin became the *lingua franca* for pharmacy in modern times.

The books were said to have been transferred as a love token by Mark Antony to Cleopatra's home land and lodged in Alexandria, as I have said before. It makes a good, happy-ever-after story, but the snag is that the transfer took place from Pergamon in 133 BC during the time of Cleopatra II and not at the time of the suzerainty of the *femme fatale* Cleopatra VII, of bathing-in-asses-milk, asp-in-the-bosom fame, which was about one hundred years later. Whatever the full story, it is known that as many as 200 000 volumes were involved.

To return to Hippocrates, at least the titular head of most of the writings and his teachings. How did his methods fare in other hands after his death? The Hippocratic method was to observe all, study the patient rather than the disease, evaluate honestly and assist nature – all very laudable. More than that, though, the instructions were clear and to the point. Others who followed lacked this virtue of brevity.

For instance, Plato's thesis *Timaeus* contains long and dilated passages not only on medicine but on the nature of the human state. He muses on the parts of the soul, mortal below the neck, immortal above it. Reason was said to emanate from between the neck and the diaphragm. Rather interestingly, he theorised that the length and tortuosity of the bowel prevented rapid absorbtion of food, a constraint which, he felt, prevents us from having to eat continuously. This desirable state of affairs allows men and women time to lead a cultivated and leisured life.

Plato was undecided as to whether the brain or semen was the essential stuff of life – a somewhat sexist view and quite divorced from the actual practice of medicine on Cos and elsewhere. Indeed, the old philosopher wrote with the lofty detachment of a medical theorist who has never had to treat a child with earache in the middle of the night. Disease to him was a lack of harmony between the elements of earth, fire, air and water; discord of the humours, in fact.

He rather neatly rounds it off in his chapter of fevers, probably at that time mainly due to malaria. Seasonal fevers, he says, are due to excess air; fever every third day excess of water; every fourth day of earth; all are initiated in the first place by excess of fire. It has a guileless simplicity but, again, what about the fever of a child in the night? You cannot find the house, it's raining and, anyway, what happened to the treatment you gave to the mother yesterday?

There were many other less famous but equally dedicated writers such as Philestion, Timetheus, Abas, Dexippus and Praxagoras of Cos, and Diocles, student of Aristotle. They all contributed to the *Corpus Hippocraticum* and, while not as esoteric as Plato, were concerned with the passage of bile and phlegm and ebbing and flowing of blood to explain disease. These and other worthies kept the flag flying from the time of the death of Hippocrates in 360 BC to the next event in the history of medicine – the establishment of the Alexandria School of Medicine.

THE ALEXANDRIA SCHOOL OF MEDICINE

WHEN ALEXANDER the Great died at the age of thirty-three in 323 BC his massive empire was divided among his generals. By dint of some opportunism, Ptolemy acquired Egypt. He himself was a fine writer and historian but it was his son, Ptolemy II, born on the island of Cos, who created the scientific system of the country and who built the museum, library and other educational institutions in what is now Alexandria. By so doing he attracted the great scholars, theologians and physicians of the period. Of the physicians, the greatest were Herophilus and Erasistratus of Ceos.

The medical school was established in about 280 or 300 BC. The crucial difference between its workings and outlook and the theories and practice of previous schools was that dissection was not only allowed but encouraged. The library was the showpiece of the new university and at its peak contained 500 000 to 700 00 volumes. It lasted for about 600 years but, regrettably, not even its footings are now in evidence. They are buried without trace under modern Alexandria and even their exact location is uncertain.

Before the fundamentals of diagnosis and treatment can be grasped it is necessary to appreciate what the body looks like and how it works in the normal state. Up to the time of this new school,

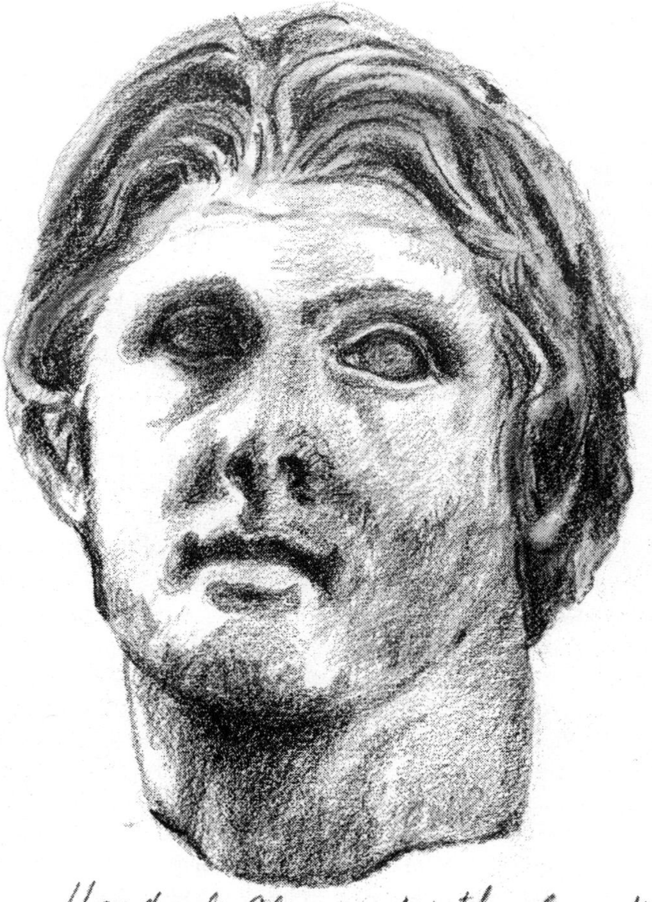

Head of Alexander the Great.

as I say, that had not been possible as the current belief was that the dead body still had some awareness and should be buried whole. Now new ideas were being bandied about and the faculty comprising Herophilus and his colleagues took advantage of the updated rules.

The snag was that in their eagerness the anatomists and trainee surgeons did not confine themselves to the dead but had a perchance to carve up the living as well. They managed to get hold of criminals and the so-called insane and, on the age old pretext of serving the greater ends of mankind and the common good, coolly went about their grisly business.

Whatever moral objections people may have held, great advances in the understanding of anatomy and physiology were made. And however squeamish we may feel, the results passed permanently into medical thinking. The same could not happen today, as witnessed by the fact that results of experiments on the inmates of Nazi concentration camps have been ignored by the profession.

Herophilus is credited with being the first in the Western world to measure the pulse and look inside the skull at the brain. Indeed, the descriptive words he used for the covering of that organ, *pia mater* and *dura mater*, are still with us. One can imagine the awe felt when looking into the head for the first time; it must have been akin to that of Hillary when he stood on top of Everest. Herophilus also named the duodenum, a part of the small bowel. He demonstrated his new knowledge by holding public dissection classes for the more resolute student.

Erasistratus was more concerned with what made the body work than with its structure. He had no time for the humeral theory and attributed disease to 'plethora' or an excess of blood. But he was a prophet before his time, for other even more powerful voices upheld the humeral theory and its basic idea survived for centuries after the Alexandria school had faded. He did, however, believe in the traditional thinking regarding blood circulation. This was, of course, that the arteries contained air, the veins alone containing blood. He, like everyone else, knew that the arteries bled if you severed them, but the party line was that, on cutting, the air or pneuma rushed out to leave a vacuum which was immediately filled with blood from the adjoining vein by passing through minute interconnecting vessels. Capillaries were unknown at the time.

The heart, he averred, contained pneuma on the left side and blood on the right, and each beat propelled the different media into the different vessels. It seems strange now that such a distinguished and massive intellect should miss the real explanation of blood circulation. With hindsight it appears so obvious, but that particular gobbet of information was not elucidated until Harvey came along 1600 years later.

It was Erasistratus who first noticed the difference between motor (or moving) and sensory (or feeling) nerves. Despite that, he thought that the nerves were hollow tubes filled with fluid. This grand but chancy researcher also believed that food liquified in the stomach and was thereupon forced by some unknown pressure into the liver. Once in the liver it was converted into blood. Well, sort of, I guess. But that was marginally better than Aristotle who earlier had thought that food was cooked in the stomach by body heat. I have heard of being consumed by the heat of passion, but body heat would not even keep a stew on the simmer.

Herophilus and Erasistratus worked together or, rather, at the same time for, in fact, they were rivals. Perhaps it was their desire to outdo one another that made the medical school great because it was only in their time, from about 300 to 250 BC that it really flourished. After that it was the same old story of dissenting factions with stagnation of progress and ideas. Acrimony with fights over order of precedence and other meaningless matters became more important than academic betterment and certainly more important than the treatment of patients.

Teaching and thinking became very convoluted and various philosophies – each with their devotees – arose. They not only confuse us at this distance but eventually helped speed medicine into the dark ages. The first of the new idealists to emerge were the Empirics. They led the way for other factions to sport fanciful names – the Dogmatists, the Pneumatists, the Methodists. Their doctrinaire stance lay in differences in philosophical approach rather than actual symptoms presented by the exasperated patient.

The Empirics concerned themselves with treatment only and would have nothing to do with the reasons for illness. Their success depended on what they learned from previous experience only and further study was regarded as quite superfluous as nature was not to be comprehended. They discarded single instances of disease pattern, insisting on a collection of similar happenings before a proposition could be made. That has a certain modern ring, I must admit, but it cramped the style of those who had imagination or who, on the other hand, wished to theorise without observing disease processes. Anyway, their star waned and they lost their way in a morass of conjecture.

They and their fellow armchair speculators undermined the greatness of the Alexandrian school and like the empire of Alexander itself, it faded into shadowy mythology. Nothing is left of it now, not even any of the writings of its two greatest sons. We only know of them through the works of others.

The school struggled on until about AD300 although the city had been overrun 200 years before that. But, as with most things in life, as one star faded another arose. In this case the new power was a man whose word held sway without being questioned for 500 years, and it is at Galen we look next.

GALEN

IT WAS during the time of Alexandria's greatness that Pergamon was holding a parallel course of eminence in the Old World with its Temple of Healing. Indeed, the Egyptians became so jealous of its supposed supremacy that their Pharaoh forbade the exporting of papyrus to Pergamon. Papyrus was the contemporary commodity for recording and keeping observations. The embargo effectively stopped the essential work and locals were forced to look elsewhere for writing material. Being resourceful and practical people, they quickly devised a method of adapting animal skins to replace the reeds. It was called Pergamos, or parchment, and eventually proved to be better than the original.

It was also at Pergamon, towards the end of its golden era, that one of the great medical intellects of ancient times, second only to Hippocrates, was born. He was Claudius Galen.

Galen has not the popular or folksy image of his distinguished predecessor, and his name is not so readily recognised nowadays. This is perhaps because he was not full of homely and punchy aphorisms nor worldly rubrics, but was more of a philosopher-physician. Not for him sitting under bent trees dispersing wisdom, nor even being party to the burning of old libraries. The word Galenism has not the currency of, for instance, Platonic or

Hippocratic. Despite this, it was medical biology which formed the more of his original thinking.

Galen was born in about AD130 during the reign of Hadrian, a man more concerned with keeping the Scots and Picts out of England than administering Temples of Healing at the other end of his empire. He came from a well-to-do background, his father being an architect concerned with building in the Temple area. One can imagine that he pushed young Claudius forward into what he saw as a nice little business in healing. Actually he claimed he directed the boy's path after a vision.

The young Galen received his education first from his father and later from teachers in medicine and philosophy in Smyrna and Corinth. Later still he went to Alexandria to complete his medical training before returning at the age of twenty-eight to Pergamon, ready to take on the world. He came rather closer to this vision than he fancied because his first job was as physician to the school of gladiators. There was plenty of stitching up in this position and his surgical skills became finely honed. Several years later he went to Rome by special invitation, such was the spread of his fame. He served three Emperors, including Marcus Aurelius, as personal physician. His escalating fame was partly due to these regal connections and partly due to his willingness to take on patients other doctors had pronounced incurable. He displayed an arrogance and immodesty regarding his deeds which not only alienated his fellow health professionals, which was bad enough in itself, but he compounded the irritation by usually being right.

He undertook public lectures and dissected animals, human dismemberment, of course, being forbidden. This enhanced his reputation in the public's eyes. All the while he was writing down his anatomical and clinical observations as well as his opinion of his contemporaries. Everything he did seemed designed to set him on a collision course with his colleagues. And so it came to pass, for in AD166 he left the city of Rome with unseemly haste, explaining that the snide remarks of his fellow medics were more than flesh and blood could stand. In fact, it was he himself who had thrown the stones in the capital's glass house, and it may well have been that the appearance of plague in the city was a more compelling reason to leave.

Incidentally, it was plague in 295 BC which prompted the first physician ever to go to Rome. Or so it is said. It seems the epidemic was so bad that the city fathers in their desperation sent to Epidaurus for a loan of Aescalapius himself. The god agreed but symbolically turned himself into a serpent. He boarded a boat which sailed for Rome but as the vessel went up the Tiber Aescalapius slipped from the bows and landed on a promontory where the river divides. He administered to the sick from there with great success, whereupon the grateful locals built a temple on the site with unprecedented hospital-type accommodation. It was constructed in the shape of a boat and the remains of the prow with sculptured snake are still visible.

But back to Galen who, two years after he had fled the city, was called back by Marcus Aurelius to become personal physician to his son and heir, Commodus.

Having one patient only was just what Galen wanted, for it allowed him to get on with his writings, and in their production lies his greatest fame, for eighty-three of his original volumes have survived to this day in their entirety.

Being prevented by law from dissecting human bodies, he restricted himself to pigs and monkeys, especially the Barbary ape. Nevertheless, he urged his students to be always on the lookout for the occasional human bone exposed in the graveyard. He was not above a bit of cemetery opportunism – he writes that on one occasion he found the body of an executed robber whose bones had been picked clean by predators of which, presumably, he was one.

It was primarily the monkey or ape, however, which was his source of experimentation and whilst the primates share many characteristics of humans, they are not identical, and it was because of that simple fact that he made his fundamental error. His observations were acute and accurate, particularly with muscles and bones, but he erred when he attempted to translate animal structure to humans.

Galen showed that arteries carried blood and not air, as their name implied. But he did not tumble to the fact that blood circulated through the body. He felt the liver and not the heart was the most important organ in the vascular system. Blood was formed there, he said, and carried to the periphery where it was turned into flesh. The blood passed from the left to the right side of the heart through minute pores in the dividing wall. He felt the heart was not so much a pump to drive blood as a kind of fireplace to heat it. The blood, he concluded, ebbed and flowed and both the venous and arterial systems were closed. Blood in the venous system was dark and thick because, he thought, it was rich in particles of food to provide nutrition to the body. The arterial system had a brighter, warmer and less viscous blood, characteristic of the presence of vital spirits and heat. Perhaps not a bad guess in the light of contemporary thinking. Galen also felt that somewhere in the periphery the systems 'mutually received from each other blood and spirits through certain invisible and extremely small vessels', as he put it.

Not until Malphigi in the post-Harvey era, in the seventeenth century AD, were capillaries defined. It seems odd that none of Galen's disciples took up the loose ends of his work and continued to explore the possibilities of circulation around the body.

In general, Galen's views of disease were those of Hippocrates, a man whom he held supreme. He kept himself aloof from the various trendies of the day but was street-wise enough to do a little merchandising of his skill and reputation: he collected plants with known therapeutic effects and sold them from a shop near the Forum in Rome. I imagine it would have been very lucrative for he was a great believer in this form of treatment – indeed, herbal remedies are still sometimes called Galenicals.

His basic tenet of medicine or, indeed of the human state, was that the well-being of man required equilibrium between the four humours, blood, yellow bile, black bile and phlegm, and the three pneumas of animal spirit, natural spirit and vital spirit. Galen regarded this truth as of such fundamental importance it was as though it had been passed down to him by a Supreme Being and engraved on tablets of stone. That may not be so fanciful because during his lifetime and for 1500 years after he was held as some kind of infallible divinity whose every utterance was considered to be The Word.

The question is, why was this so? How did he maintain his

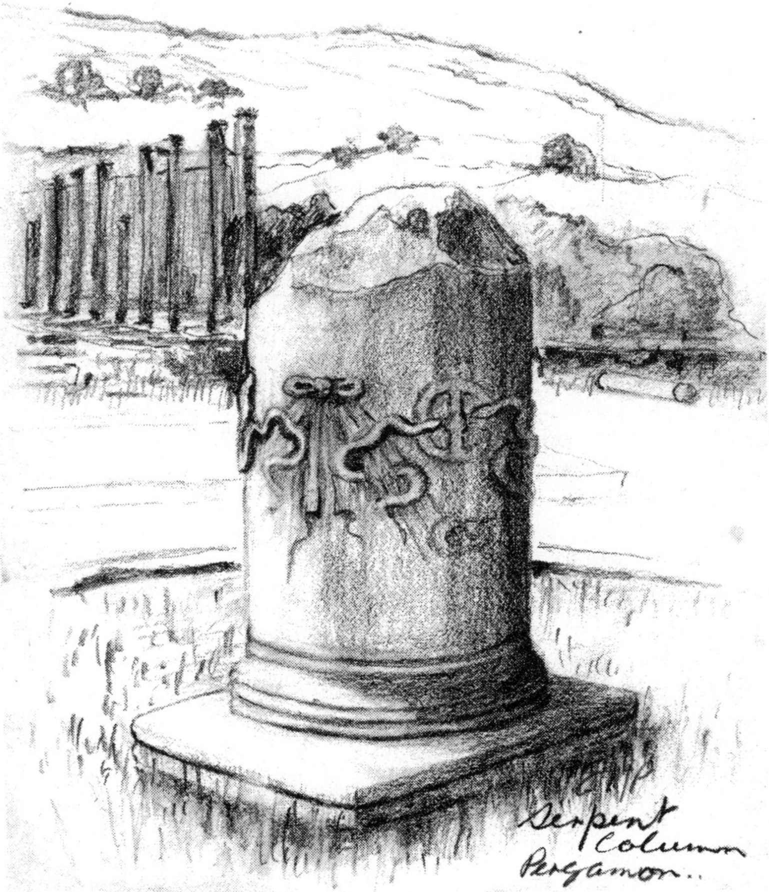

fallacious reputation for so long? Almost certainly it was due to his connection with the Church. He was a declared and avowed monotheist and firmly held that the human state consists of body and soul and of these two the soul is eternal and so more important. This kind of publicly held belief, coming from such a well known identity who enjoyed royal patronage, was exactly the kind of ex-cathedra statement the fledgling Christian Church needed in order to gain credence. It was in line with the teachings of Paul, and so Christians embraced Galen as a convert. And who can blame them? If Christianity had foundered it is quite likely we would never have heard of Galen and the course of medicine would have taken a different direction.

It is true that Galen wrote of Moses and of Christ, but whether he was in fact a convert is not certain. As it happened, his spiritual beliefs fitted other contemporary religions equally well, but as Christianity claimed him, it also claimed as its own his philosophy and writings. As Christians became more entrenched as a major force, the Church decided what could be published and what could not, thus censoring unfavourable comment. Being a believer, and so a favourite son, Galen received the ecclesiastical stamp of approval and his books and their multiple errors became Canon law. The result is that not only have eighty-three of Galen's fully authenticated works survived until today, having been preserved in theological libraries, but medical progress was plunged into a therapeutic Dark Age.

Whilst it may have been a thin period for medical research, the advent of Christianity did at least provide the impetus for the development of another feature of medicine which has survived up to today. This was the establishment of hospitals. The Temples of Healing of ancient Greece were not built out of compassion for the sick, and were not hospitals in the caring sense with which we associate them today. Their functions were more comparable to a contemporary trip to Lourdes with its chance of a miracle cure. With Christianity came philosophies such as universal love, being your brother's keeper, emulating the good Samaritan, helping the needy and similar benevolent attitudes which naturally led to caring establishments or hospitals. The very first example of this principle was on that island in the Tiber at Rome, but that was a one-off event and, anyway, was a modified temple. It did not become a way of life until the early centuries after Christ.

Besides his books on clinical observations and practice, Galen also wrote on philosophy. He was, to put it kindly, somewhat wordy, and so his works have been largely shied away from. It is said that, having once written a book, he was a great man for second thoughts, and his supplements not infrequently surpassed the length of the original. This prolixity was reflected in his social intercourse for a biographer said of him, 'He showed his teeth when laughing, talked much, and was rarely silent'. I can well imagine it.

Galen was a keen admirer of Aristotle and accepted his notions of the elements and the purposeful workings of Nature. But he disagreed on basic biological questions such as the seat of the soul, the relative function of the brain, heart, liver, and on some questions of space and time. For instance, Galen deemed that everything that moves something else must necessarily itself be moved. But he accepted the Aristotelian view that 'Nature does nothing in vain', and sought to show that organic structure such as the bones and muscles of the hand serve the function for which they were designed. Who or what designed it in the first place, whether a Divine Creator or just a munificent nature, Galen was not clear.

In AD192 a great fire in the district of the Temple of Peace in Rome destroyed many unique manuscripts of his writing. Even so, about 1200 pages of script remain.

The exact date and place of his death are not known, but he left a legacy of dominance unique in medical history. As Osler was to say of him about one hundred years ago, 'For fifteen centuries he dominated medical thought as powerfully as did Aristotle in the schools. Not until the Renaissance did daring spirits begin to question the infallibility of the medical Pope'.

CELSUS AND ROMAN MEDICINE

BETWEEN THE eras of Hippocrates and Galen, in a time span of about 500 years, there existed a number of medical ideologies which had the support of a series of enthusiastic physicians. Scraps of their fervour have filtered down to us but, apart from the dons at Alexandria, none made far-reaching conclusions nor caught our imagination. Most of the medical thinking, such as it was, was undertaken in the Eastern Mediterranean around the traditional sites. But at almost exactly the time of Christ there lived in Rome a man who provided a brilliant exception to the dominance of medicine by the Greeks.

Not only was he not Greek, he was not even medically trained and, more than that, he was a man of noble birth who dabbled in what his contemporaries regarded as the messy and degrading activitites of a profession which in Rome was the province of slaves and other inferior riff-raff. Because of all this his eventual acceptance by the medical fraternity was remarkable and he sealed his pre-eminence by writing a book in about AD30. This was not any old book but a treatise which survives today as the *non-pareil* in its description of the era – the definitive work.

The name of this paragon was Aulus Cornelius Celsus.

Celsus was a man of culture and broad interest, as befitted a member of the leisured and wealthy classes. He was equally at ease expanding on philosophy, law, military strategy and rhetoric, and contemplating the diseased state. Although we know he wrote on all these subjects, only his works on medicine have survived as the Book 1 to Book 8 of *De Medicina*.

Celsus was born during the empire of Tiberius in about 25 BC and lived to become famous enough to be written about by such well-known Roman eulogists as Pliny the Elder and Quintilian. Indeed, he was dubbed the Cicero of medicine.

De Medicina was written, naturally enough, in Latin and set out what Celsus considered to be the best medical practices of the day. As such it is a unique historical document for he drew on traditions of the Hellenistic School as well as contemporary Roman ideas. Charges of being a copyist compiler can and have been hurled against him. But if he was a copier he was an honest copier, if there is such a thing. Also, he brought current thoughts under one cover and allowed the Roman physicians to get some accuracy, order and consistency into their work. The theories and aphorisms may not have been his, but they are the only ones we have and, after two thousand years, who is counting anyway?

Many of the conclusions have a remarkably modern flavour. For instance, he espoused the idea that the patient should be considered as a whole and not just be regarded as the interesting thyroid or stomach or big toe in Ward 2, so to speak. This type of de-personalisation has been a grouch against doctors for centuries. Having established that, he goes on, '. . .and, therefore, since the acquaintance of both (ie patient and disease) by the physician should be equally emphasised, it is more useful that the physician be a friend rather than a stranger. I believe the medical art should be rational and gain instruction from evident causes, and with all obscure causes rejected from the art but not from the reflection of the skilled physician'.

Celsus was keen on health habits. He wrote that people who have been occupied during the day, '. . .should take exercise which ought always to precede the eating of food. The exercise should be ampler for him who has laboured less and digested well, and it should be lighter for him who is tired and who has thought less during the day.' That sounds reasonable enough and he goes on to point out that useful exercises included drill, hand ball, walking and reading aloud. Presumably this last is to exercise the larynx of the quiet achiever. The various activities should be continued, he averred, until sweating occurred, 'or at any rate lassitude, which should be well this side of fatigue'.

He seems to have had a laconic style which has lost nothing in the translation. Besides being succinct, his *bon mots* display tact, wisdom and a homely common-sense. The whole makes compelling reading.

Take, for instance, his considered opinion on the place of sexual intercourse in the grand scheme of life. 'Sexual intercourse' he says, 'neither should be avidly desired, nor should it be feared very much. Rarely performed it revives the body, performed frequently it weakens. However, since nature and not number should be considered in frequency, together with age and state of body, sexual union is recognised as not harmful when it is followed by neither apathy nor pain.'

The writings of Celsus demonstrate the pragmatic approach of the Romans to health, and many illustrate the strong tradition of family self-help which they developed. In the Empire at that time the head of the household in the more socially disadvantaged families took the role of medical consultant as well as bread-winner. In the upper and more wealthy echelons, a Greek slave was employed to oversee the various ailments of staff and family, for it was well-known that Greeks had some basic medical training.

That, of course, may have been all very well for the bellicose and insensitive Romans, but the Greek practitioners of the Eastern Mediterranean did not care to be confused with their countrymen in menial positions, however facile with the physic, so they were somewhat contemptuous of those who were associated with them, including Celsus. So this, plus the fact that his book was written in Latin and not Greek, the *lingua franca* of contemporary science, led to *De Medicina* being generally ignored by them. As at that time they were all powerful in such matters, the book fell into obscurity.

And so it would have remained but for its fortunate discovery 1400 years later. Where it had been all that time is unclear, but it turned up in the Vatican where Pope Nicholas V (1397-1455) recognised both its historical and its practical worth. By happy chance its resurfacing coincided with the development of a new skill – the use of moveable type in printing. So in 1478 *De Medicina* was printed in Florence to become the first medical tract set up on the new-fangled technology. Since then many editions have been run off, and it can be found in all respectable medical libraries. Its first English edition came out in 1756.

Out of the eight books, several classic passages have emerged which are still bandied about by the more pompous of the medical profession today. Let me give you a few examples. Of blood letting Celsus has this to say, '. . .it is very easy to one who has experience, yet very difficult to one who is ignorant, for the veins lie near to the arteries and to those the nerves'. Hardly a unique contribution to the sum total of human knowledge, but one which is regularly resurrected by those in authority when addressing the new graduates. I bet they do not know where it originated.

In the third book the so-called 'blood fevers' are discussed. The usual cause of sweating fever in Rome at that time was malaria, but the author recounts more reasons such as jaundice, consumption and other infectious diseases. It is in this volume that the famous and succinct description of inflammation appears. It is still drummed into medical students in its original Latin – Calor, Rubor, Tumor and Dolor, or heat, redness, swelling and pain. If you think of a boil or infected tonsils that description cannot be bettered.

Book Six is given over to diseases of the ear, eye, skin and teeth. To remove a foreign body from some unfortunate's ear, it is recommended that the patient is bound to a board which is fixed to the normal side. He or she is then made to lie down with the board uppermost and the afflicted ear to the ground. The timber is then brought a smart blow with a previously concealed hammer. The author simply concludes, 'What is within the ear drops out.' Let's hope that is all which does drop out.

Book Seven contains the well-known ideal of the perfect surgeon. In passing, the parsing of surgeon is always, I fear, in the masculine. But, right or wrong, that was the way of the world then as, indeed, it seems to be now. The homily goes, 'He should be youthful, or at any rate nearer to youth than to older age; with a strong and healthy hand which never trembles, and ready to use the left hand as well as the right; with sharp vision and clear; and with spirit undaunted; filled with pity, so that he wishes to cure the patient yet is not moved by his cries to go too fast or cut less than necessary; but he does everything just as if the cries of pain cause him no emotion.' The advent of anaesthesia in the last 150 years has made parts of that definition redundant, but I would still like to think a surgeon needs a steady hand and sharp vision.

It is also in this book that Celsus gives details of the trick needed to remove arrow heads, to repair hernias or remove a bladder stone. He also gives a remarkably modern description of how to remove tonsils by shelling them out with the fingers. Splints for fractures are described, as are bandages stiffened with starch to facilitate rigidity. Celsus had a sublime mastery of illness, its various causes, its natural history and its treatment within the limits of contemporary understanding. Medicine at that time was a specialised segment within the broad field of traditional philosophy. Unlike the attitudes of the Egyptians and their predecessors who looked on illness in magical and therapeutically empirical terms, the Greeks and Romans, as we have seen, thought of it in global or conceptual terms.

One particular area where the Romans shone was in the field of public health. They may have contributed little in diagnosis and treatment, but their system of sanitation and water supply was unequalled. Rome itself was surrounded by marshes and these were drained in Etruscan times. A little later, in the sixth century BC, the main sewer or *Cloaca Maxima* was constructed and was the exit into the Tiber of an elaborate system of pipes under the city.

Until about the third century BC the river Tiber was the only source of drinking water for Rome, but then construction of the famous aqueducts was begun. They conveyed water to the city from miles around. By the first century BC, there were nine such water channels and the water was purified by being allowed to stand in settling basins along the route. At the beginning of the Christian era there were fourteen aqueducts supplying about 250 litres a day per head of population. Eventually many others were built throughout their conquered territory. Such an abundance of water, of course, allowed for domestic and civic fountains, swimming pools, public baths and gymnasia as well as ample drinking water. The Romans may not have been very talented in medical science, but they always presented as clean patients.

Reference has already been made to the establishment of the first hospital in Rome when Aescalapius, masquerading as a snake stepped ashore on an island in the Tiber. That hospital was mainly used for the treatment of slaves, sent there to avoid the trouble of caring for them at home, so it became a haven for the sick poor.

Being a belligerent people, however, the Romans made sure the military were cared for and medical men were part of the army's establishment. Although ranked as non-commissioned officers, no good letting them get ideas above their station, they were exempt from taxation and combat duties. On Trajan's column, still to be seen in Rome, is sculptured a scene showing the workings of what looks like a first-aid dressing station. Military hospitals were established at various strategic points along the army's lines of communication throughout Europe.

Despite their public health and legionary medicine, the Romans, as we have seen, were not well-known for their therapeutic excellence. Indeed, endemic malaria in the capital undermined the mental and physical well-being of the population to such a degree that it was probably a major factor in the eventual demise

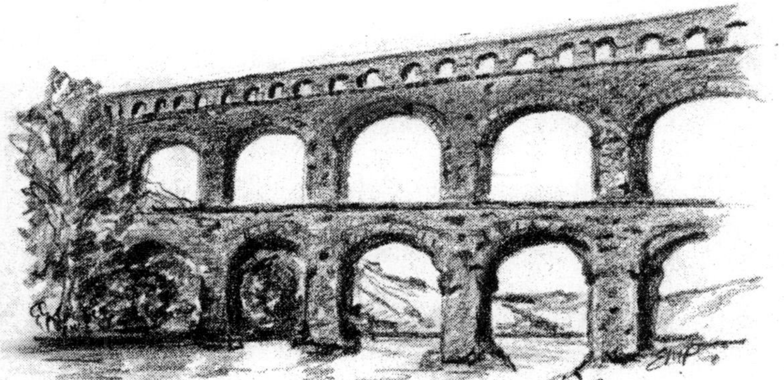

Roman aqueduct.
at Nimes.

of the Empire. Their place in medical history is more assured by the writings of Celsus then by clinical acumen, and it is he who should have the final mention.

Celsus, and a little later Galen, between them wrote the most complete medical encyclopaedia of the classical world. For his part, Celsus stated the facts and refrained from indulging in specious argument and theory. Galen, on the other hand, presented as a kind of medical dictator and his fame is based on investigations and experiment rather than clinical work. Both had their place but the caring nature and home-spun advice of Celsus gives him a greater human appeal than probably anyone in the ancient world.

In any event, when these two disappeared from the scene a kind of clinical Dark Age descended on the art and practice of medicine and little was added to the pool of knowledge for almost 1500 years. Then, in 1526, the irascible Paracelsus not only questioned the great Galen but also burnt his books as so much prehistoric rubbish. In 1540, Versalius defied long convention and dissected a human body in detail for the first time and agreed with Paracelsus.

That was the end of the old order which had started in prehistory and progressed through Mesopotamia, India, China, Egypt, Greece and Rome. It had lasted with little major change for thousands of years, but then it was questioned as never before and the flood-gates were opened. The ways of Marduk, Dhanvantari, Imhotep, Aescalapius, other gods of healing and their earthly disciples were over forever.